☞ T5-AVO-801

DISCARDED BY

MACPHÁIDÍN LIBRARY

MACPHÁIDÍN LIBRARY
STONEHILL COLLEGE
EASTON, MASSACHUSETTS 02357

# Understanding Chronic Pain

Understanding Health and Sickness Series
*Miriam Bloom, Ph.D.*
*General Editor*

# Understanding Chronic Pain

**Angela J. Koestler, Ph.D.**
**Ann Myers, M.D.**

University Press of Mississippi
Jackson

www.upress.state.ms.us

Copyright © 2002 by University Press of Mississippi
All rights reserved
Manufactured in the United States of America
Illustrations by Karen Wing
10  09  08  07  06  05  04  03  02    4  3  2  1
∞

Library of Congress Cataloging-in-Publication Data

Koestler, Angela J.
    Understanding chronic pain / Angela J. Koestler, Ann Myers.
        p. cm.—(Understanding health and sickness series)
    Includes index.
    ISBN 1-57806-439-2 (cloth : alk. paper)—ISBN 1-57806-440-6 (paper : alk.
paper)
    1. Chronic pain—Popular works. [DNLM: 1. Pain—therapy—Popular
Works. 2. Chronic Disease—therapy—Popular Works. WL 704 K78U
2002] I. Myers, Ann. II. Title. III. Series.
RB127 .K645 2002
616'.0472—dc21                                                    2002001017

British Library Cataloging-in-Publication Data available

Pain—has an Element of Blank—
It cannot recollect
When it begun—or if there were
A time when it was not—

—Emily Dickinson

# Contents

# Acknowledgments

We are indebted to Dr. Lee Giffin and Dr. Sandra Burford, who are family medicine physicians, for taking time out of their busy schedules to review this manuscript and offer their valuable suggestions. We also extend thanks to the following individuals for their support and suggestions throughout the writing of this book: Annette Hitt, Dr. Rahul Vohra (medical director of Methodist Rehabilitation Center), Helen Wright, Dr. Robert Kores, Wanda King, Tammy Beard, Dr. Billye Bob Currie, Dr. Katherine Nordal, Dr. Ben Root, Dr. Elizabeth Henderson, Dr. Sharon Pugh, Dr. Pat Ainsworth, Dr. Ann Wheeless, Evelyn Knight Price, and our friends and families. And last, but most important, our thanks go out to the patients we serve.

This book is dedicated to the memory of Pauline O'Hara and Patricia Dickerson.

# Introduction

Illness is the doctor to whom we pay most heed; to kindness, to knowledge, we make promise only; pain we obey.

—Marcel Proust, *Remembrance of Things Past*

Chronic pain has been a cause of human suffering from the beginning of time. Stories about pain and its devastating consequences on the quality of human life have been recorded throughout history. Reference is made to King Ra in ancient Egypt who had bouts of severe head pain. In 1683 English physician Thomas Sydenham described the pain he had suffered from gout for thirty-four years. During the Civil War many surgeons wrote of the pain and suffering experienced by wounded soldiers, who, after amputation, were left with phantom limb pain. Sigmund Freud wrote about the effects of cancer pain after he was diagnosed with cancer of the jaw. Today, the medical literature is filled with examples of people who are left with chronic pain following an injury and the effects the pain has on the quality of their lives. Chronic pain can affect our ability to function in our jobs and can prevent us from participating in many activities that we once enjoyed. It affects relationships with our families, friends, coworkers, and employers. Chronic pain can be debilitating physically, emotionally, socially, and financially, and, unfortunately, it is not uncommon.

In the United States approximately 90 million people suffer from a chronic pain condition, with an estimated cost exceeding $125 billion annually in health care costs, disability compensation, lost productivity, and tax revenue. Chronic pain disables more people than cancer or heart disease and costs us more than both combined. It is estimated that 5 million Americans are partially disabled by back problems, and another 2 million are so severely disabled that they cannot work. Twenty million people suffer from arthritis pain, 40 million experience chronic recurrent headaches, and the majority of individuals in intermediate or advanced stages of cancer suffer moderate to severe pain.

Only within the last two decades has there been a surge of interest in specifically addressing the issue of chronic pain and its relief through research and clinical application. Previously, it was believed that pain was necessarily associated with tissue damage. Pain that persisted past the normal time of healing was discounted and attributed to neurosis or hysteria. Over the last twenty years our understanding of the underlying mechanisms of chronic pain has significantly increased. It is now recognized that many factors contribute to the experience of pain besides actual tissue damage, and chronic pain can persist beyond the normal time of healing. Chronic pain is a multidimensional phenomenon that involves physiological, psychological, and social factors.

Chronic pain is no longer treated as a symptom, but as a specific medical problem to be addressed with specific treatment modalities and interventions. In most patients with chronic conditions such as back disorders and arthritis, it is not the underlying pathology but pain that interferes with functioning and the quality of patients' lives. Even with the strides made in recent years, our basic understanding of chronic pain remains limited. For example, with rheumatoid arthritis, the immediate cause of the pain is known, but the reasons why the disease causes pain are not clearly understood. At present, there is no cure for chronic pain.

Pain accounts for more than 35 million new office visits and more than 70 million of all office visits to physicians each year in the United States. Although there is no cure for chronic pain, there are effective treatment models that focus on the management of pain and quality of life issues. A multi-disciplinary team approach that involves physician specialists, psychologists, physical therapists, and other health care practitioners is one of the more effective models for the treatment of chronic pain. This model takes into consideration the multifactorial nature of the chronic pain phenomenon and emphasizes the patient's involvement in the treatment process.

Our purpose here is to provide information about the mechanisms of chronic pain and about current treatment approaches; this book is intended for those individuals who suffer from a chronic pain condition, as well as for their families, coworkers, employers, and friends. Chronic pain remains a major challenge for those who suffer from it and for health care professionals and scientists who continue to seek more effective treatments and, ultimately, a cure.

We begin the book with a brief overview of the conceptualization and treatment of chronic pain throughout history and conclude the first chapter with current definitions of chronic pain and its impact on the individual and society. In chapter 2, we examine the causes of chronic pain by reviewing underlying mechanisms, theoretical models, and factors that affect pain. We then identify pain treatment specialists and discuss their role in the treatment process. Treatment approaches that are discussed include medications, physical intervention (e.g., surgery and spinal blocks), physical rehabilitation, and psychological interventions. Next, we emphasize the patient's role in the treatment process and the assumption of self-care responsibilities. Information is provided on how pain sufferers can begin to take control of their pain by using cognitive and behavioral strategies, while complying with medical treatment recommendations. Learning how to identify factors that increase and decrease pain sensations is an important component in the self-management of pain and suffering.

Chapters 5, 6, 7, 8, and 9 are devoted to reviewing specific pain conditions and current treatment approaches. Topics of discussion include back pain, neuropathic pain, rheumatic pain, cancer pain, headaches, interstitial cystitis, and sickle cell disease. Obviously, there are many chronic pain conditions that we do not address in this book, but we attempt to provide basic information about the management of pain that is applicable to most chronic pain conditions. In the final chapter, we discuss current research efforts and the movement toward finding more effective treatment methods and a cure for chronic pain.

We used many sources during the writing of this book, consulting publications by John Bonica, Ronald Melzack, Patrick Wall, Dennis Turk, David Tollison, Wilbert Fordyce, Richard Sternbach, Gerald Aronoff, and others. Additional references included publications by the American Pain Society and International Association for the Study of Pain. Last, and most important, we consulted the patients with whom we work. Unless we suffer from chronic pain ourselves, we can gain an understanding of the experience of pain only through those who bear its burden day after day after day.

# Understanding Chronic Pain

# I. What Is Chronic Pain?

It is easier to find men who will volunteer to die, than to find those who are willing to endure pain with patience.

—Julius Caesar

The search for a cure for pain and pain-relieving techniques is not a new endeavor. References to pain and pain interventions are recorded on Babylonian clay tablets that date from 2250 b.c.e. From the beginning of humankind, we have sought ways to alleviate pain and suffering. Through the centuries our view of the causes of pain and the center of pain sensation has changed, but many pain-relieving techniques used by early peoples are used today. With the technological advances of the twentieth century, we have taken those original ideas and shaped them into more effective treatments and interventions. However, often the basic premise remains the same. In surveying previous eras and cultures, it becomes obvious that we continue to address similar questions in our search for a cure for pain. What causes pain? What are the underlying mechanisms of pain? What eliminates or reduces pain and suffering? To gain a perspective on how and why we arrived at our present conceptualization of chronic pain and treatment methodology, we must examine the evolution of our theories and their application to pain and suffering.

## History of Pain

Primitive cultures thought pain was caused by magical fluids or by intrusions of evil spirits or demons. Treatments

**Table I.I. Approaches to pain in primitive cultures.**

*Intervention*

- Pressure on affected area
- Rubbing affected area
- Cold water (rivers)
- Heat (sun/fire)
- Draining fluids by excision
- Trephine of the skull
- Shock from electric fish (torpedo fish)
- Herbal potions
- Opium
- Poultices
- Physical exercise
- Prayer
- Chanting

*Prevention*

- Amulets
- Tattoos
- Rings in the ear
- Rings in the nostril
- Burning of incense
- Prayer
- Building temples and shrines

included placing pressure on the afflicted area, rubbing it, and exposing it to the cold water of rivers, to the heat of the sun, or to fire (table I.I). It was considered important to rid the sufferer of the evil spirit causing the pain. A priestess, sorceress, or, later in history, a shaman was enlisted to exorcize the demon. The medicine man sometimes inflicted small wounds in the patient to allow the evil spirits and bad fluids to escape, or he sucked the fluid out of the painful area. Herbal concoctions and healing potions were also used to ease pain. Prevention is not a new idea—amulets, talismans, tatoos, and rings in the ear or nostril were used to ward off pain-causing evil spirits.

Shrines were built in ancient Egypt to appease the gods, because pain was thought to be caused by gods or spirits of the dead which entered the body through the ear or nostril. Remedies for pain included exercise, heat, cold, and massage. Headaches were treated with surgical methods such as trephine of the skull, which involved boring a hole in the skull. Shocks from electric fish and torpedo fish were used for treatment of neuralgia, headaches, and other pain problems. The heart was thought to be the center of sensation and, therefore, of pain.

Around 500 B.C.E. in India, the Buddha attributed pain to the frustration of desires. Pain was recognized as a sensation, but the focus was on the emotional level of the experience. Joy and pain were experienced in the heart, which was considered the seat of consciousness. Also, acupuncture was being used in China to restore balance and eliminate disease. It was believed that a vital energy called the chi circulated in all parts of the body through a network of fourteen channels connected to vital organs and functions. A deficiency or excess in circulation of the chi caused an imbalance in the system and resulted in pain. Moxibustion (burning of incense), massage, physical exercise, and dietary regimens were also used as pain remedies.

In ancient Greece (third to fifth centuries B.C.E.) Alcmaeon, Plato, Aristotle, Hippocrates, Theophrastus, Herophilus, and Erasistratus were but a few who contributed to later theories about pain and pain mechanisms. Alcmaeon asserted that the brain and not the heart was the center of sensation. Some support for this theory was provided by Hippocrates, Theophrastus, Herophilus, and Erasistratus. Hippocrates considered the brain to be the center of thought and perhaps of sensation. He thought that pain arose from an excess or deficiency in one of the four humors—blood, phlegm, yellow bile, and black bile. Herophilus and Erasistratus provided anatomic evidence that the brain was part of the nervous system. They believed two types of nerves were attached to the neuroaxis. One nerve type was for movement and the other for feeling. However, these advanced ideas were over-shadowed by Plato and Aristotle, who both advocated that pain was felt in the heart as a quality or passion of the soul. The heart, they thought, was the center of sensory perception. Plato wrote that sensation resulted from the movement of atoms communicating through the veins to the heart and liver. Pain arose not only from peripheral stimulation but as an emotional experience in the soul that resided in the heart. Both pain and pleasure, although opposites, were thought to originate in the heart. Although Aristotle's writings in biology do not stand up to scrutiny, he did contribute to the understanding of sensation by distinguishing the five senses: vision, hearing, taste, smell, and touch.

During this era a transition occurred in the idea of the cause of pain. There was a shift from thinking that evil spirits caused pain to the idea that the commitment of sin brought subsequent punishment by an offended deity. The shaman or medicine man was replaced by the priest, who was considered a servant of the gods. He used natural remedies, prayers, and sacrifices to appease the gods and have them grant relief to the sufferer. Even Hippocrates alluded to this idea of pain as he stated, "Divine is the work to subdue pain." The same concept of sin and punishment was adopted in the Judeo-Christian ethic. Having eaten the forbidden apple, Eve was exiled from the garden and made to bear pain during child-birth. The fundamental significance of the word "pain" in English is derived from the Latin word "poena," meaning punishment. Subsequently, Catholicism emphasized the allevi-ation of pain by its clergy through prayer.

Throughout primitive and ancient civilizations analgesic agents were used that were derived from plants such as the poppy, mandragora, hemp, and henbane. The first written records of the use of analgesia are those contained in ancient Babylonian clay tablets. Reference is made to a cement of henbane seeds mixed with gum mastic that was applied to a cavity in the tooth as a remedy for dental pain. In ancient Egypt opium was used for the treatment of headaches and was prescribed by Isis for King Ra, who suffered with bouts of severe head pain. There are also references to the use of analgesics in Homer's *The Iliad* and *The Odyssey*. Hippocrates attributed narcotic action to a substance called mecon that most likely contained opium.

Approximately four centuries later in Rome, Galen (131 ca.–200 C.E.) discovered the central nervous system. He clearly described the anatomy of the cranial and spinal nerves, linking their function with the brain. He described three kinds of nerves: soft nerves had a sensory function, hard nerves had a motor function, and other nerves involved pain sensation. It should be noted, however, that the Aristotelian concept of pain arising in the heart as a passion of the soul prevailed for twenty-three centuries.

In the Middle Ages there was some movement toward the idea that the brain was the center of sensory perception, but it was also thought that the brain had the capacity to cool the heart. During the Renaissance period great advances were made in chemistry, physics, physiology, and anatomy. Leonardo da Vinci believed that the center of sensation was located in the third ventricle (small cavity) in the brain and that the spinal cord served as a conductor that transmitted sensations to the brain. However, during this period there were no advances in pain therapy with the exception of the somniferant sponge. The sponge was saturated with opium, mandragora, and other plants to produce drowsiness during surgery. This technique induced a deep sleep and often resulted in the death of the patient.

In 1628 when William Harvey discovered the circulation of blood, the idea that the heart was the center of sensation was still generally accepted. Later Descartes considered the brain the seat of sensation and motor function. His ideas were published in his book *De Homine* (*On Man*) in 1664, fourteen years after his death.

The eighteenth and nineteenth centuries brought about much progress in the understanding of the nervous system and the treatment of pain. Joseph Priestly discovered nitrous oxide, which led to a new era of analgesia. In 1806 morphine was isolated from crude opium, and in 1828 salicin was isolated from willow bark, which led to the development of aspirin. In 1846 Morton discovered the anesthetic properties of ether. The needle and syringe were developed. Additionally, Sigmund Freud and Carl Koller demonstrated the anesthetic efficacy of cocaine for surgical and nonsurgical pain. Nonsurgical pain was also treated with hypnosis and psychotherapeutic methods. Neurosurgical operations were performed on areas of the brain and specific nerve pathways thought to be generating pain or causing the perception of pain. Other pain treatments included electrotherapy, hydrotherapy, thermotherapy, and mechanotherapy. In the late 1800s Roentgen discovered x-rays, which led to the use of radiation for many painful conditions such as tumors.

The modern scientific study of pain actually began in the first half of the nineteenth century, when physiology emerged as an experimental science. Several theories on the nature of pain arose during this period, and by the end of the century there existed three conflicting ideas. The specificity theory stated that pain was specific sensation with its own sensory apparatus independent of touch and other senses. The intensive theory suggested that every sensory stimulus could produce pain if it reached sufficient intensity. This theory led to later concepts of pain such as the patterned theory and summation theory. The Aristotelian concept that pain was an affective (emotional) quality still prevailed among some scientists and philosophers.

There was such an intense conflict among those investigating pain and sensation that in 1885 the president of the American Psychological Association attempted to reconcile the opposing views. He suggested that pain consisted of the original sensation and the psychic reaction or displeasure provoked by the sensation. As a result, this concept was embraced by later researchers who believed that pain consisted of both sensory (body physical) and affective (emotional) dimensions.

During the first half of the twentieth century, research on pain continued, and the published data acquired were used to support either the specificity theory or the intensive theory or a modification of these. These theories served as the basis for pain treatment until in 1947 a multidisciplinary pain center was established by John Bonica, an anesthesiologist, at Tacoma General Hospital in Tacoma, Washington. He had worked in pain control at an army hospital in 1944. In treating some of his patients he began to recognize the complexity and multifactorial nature of the pain experience. Initially he formed a collaborative relationship with an orthopedist, a neurosurgeon, and a psychiatrist, and that later led to the establishment of a pain center. The clinic was moved to the University of Washington in 1960. Another multidisciplinary pain clinic was established at the University of Oregon by William K. Livingston, a surgeon. He also had been involved in the treatment and management of pain with a multidisciplinary team during World War II. In 1965 a psychologist, Ronald Melzack, and a physiologist, Patrick Wall, proposed the gate control theory of pain, which reinforced the idea of a team approach to the treatment of pain. This theory, which will be explained more fully in the next chapter, proposed that chronic pain rarely has a single cause, but is, instead, the result of several interacting causes. Although some deficiencies have been found in the anatomical and physiological aspects of this theory, it serves as a milestone in pain research and treatment, for it prompted a significant increase in pain research and directly affected our approach to pain treatment. Clinicians and scientists began to organize a movement toward the acceptance of pain as a medical problem.

The initial meeting of the International Association for the Study of Pain (IASP) was held in 1973. This organization endorses the concept of interdisciplinary collaboration and promotes pain education, research, and improved pain management. The American Pain Society (APS), which is the U.S. chapter of IASP, was formed in 1977. The APS promotes increased funding for pain research and encourages the recognition of pain as a medical problem in the United States. There are also regional chapters of APS, such as the Southern Pain Society (SPS), which encourage the establishment of local or state pain societies.

### Definition of Pain

The definition of pain most widely accepted by pain specialists was proposed by the International Association for the Study of Pain and published in the journal *Pain* in 1979. The development of this definition, along with a taxonomy of pain terminology, provides a common language for the different disciplines involved in the research and treatment of pain. This definition is as follows:

> Pain. An unpleasant sensory and emotional experience associated with actual or potential tissue damage or described in terms of such damage.
>
> Note: Pain is always subjective. Each individual learns the application of the word through experiences related to injury in early life. Biologists recognize that stimuli that cause pain are likely to damage tissue. Accordingly, pain is the experience

that we associate with actual or potential tissue damage. It is unquestionably a sensation in part or parts of the body, but it is also always unpleasant and therefore also an emotional experience. Experiences that resemble pain (e.g., pricking) but are not unpleasant should not be called pain. Unpleasant abnormal experiences (dysesthesiae) may also be pain but are not necessarily so because, subjectively, they may not have the usual sensory qualities of pain.

Many people report pain in the absence of tissue damage or any likely pathophysiologic cause; usually this happens for psychologic reasons. There is no way to distinguish their experience from that due to tissue damage if one takes the subjective report. If they regard their experience as pain and if they report it in the same ways as pain caused by tissue damage, it should be accepted as pain. This definition avoids tying pain to the stimulus. Activity induced in the nociceptor and nociceptive pathways [sensory receptors that respond to pain] by a noxious stimulus is not pain, which is always a psychologic state, even though pain most often has a proximate physical cause.

There are generally two types of pain, acute and chronic. Acute pain and chronic pain are defined separately because there are differences between the two in regard to cause, mechanisms, pathophysiology, symptomatology, biologic function, and approach to diagnosis and treatment. Generally speaking, pain is our body's alarm system. It tells us that something is wrong. When part of our body is injured or hurt, nerves in that area release chemical signals. Other nerves send these signals to our brain, where they are recognized as pain. Pain often tells us that we need to do something. For example, if we touch a hot furnace, pain signals from our brain make us pull our hand away. This type of pain helps protect us.

Acute pain is pain of recent onset and short duration. This type of pain is generally quickly diagnosed. With appropriate treatment the underlying problem is corrected and the pain is resolved. Examples of medical problems that involve acute pain are appendicitis, toothache, and fractures. The patient plays a relatively small role in determining the outcome of the problem and is generally expected to be passive and compliant in the recovery process. Psychological and environmental factors do not have as significant an influence on acute pain as they do on the chronic pain experience.

Chronic pain is pain that is ongoing and has lasted six months or longer. It is pain that has not responded to traditional medical interventions, or one for which a medical "cure" is not available. It is also defined as pain that persists a month beyond the usual course of an acute disease or a reasonable time for an injury to heal. Chronic pain can be associated with a chronic pathologic process that causes continuous pain or pain that recurs at intervals for months or years. With this type of pain the emphasis changes from finding a diagnosis and cure to rehabilitation and minimization of the negative effects of the painful condition. This is an important difference between chronic pain and acute pain, because it shifts some responsibility for management of the physical problem from health care providers to the patient. It also directs the focus of treatment away from the underlying cause of the pain to the pain itself and the lifestyle disruption it creates. Pain is no longer just a symptom; pain is the problem. Typically, this type of pain is not a useful pain, in that it does not serve as an alarm system, alerting us that something is wrong. Our understanding of chronic pain and how it affects us will be further discussed in the next chapter as we review current theoretical models and pain mechanisms. We will begin to explore the anatomical and physiological mechanisms of chronic pain and to see why the experience of chronic pain, unlike acute pain, is significantly influenced by psychological and environmental factors.

# 2. What Causes Chronic Pain?

Beauty cannot disguise nor music melt
A pain undiagnosable but felt.
—Anne Lindbergh, "The Stone," *The Unicorn and Other Poems*

Chronic pain is caused by active disease processes, tissue damage, and other insults to our body. Rheumatoid arthritis, cancer, musculoskeletal problems, cardiac disease, and headache are but a few of the conditions that can lead to chronic pain. Although science has made great advancements in its understanding of the underlying neurophysiological, anatomical, and chemical mechanisms of this complex phenomenon, much remains unknown. Many people suffer from chronic pain for which the underlying cause is unknown or the level of their suffering is considered in excess of identified pathology or disease process. These missing pieces from the puzzle prevent us from integrating all we have learned and hinder our generating a cure for chronic pain conditions.

How do we go about finding these missing pieces? Our understanding of the causes of chronic pain begins with theoretical models. Theoretical models integrate experimental and clinical observations into a system that provides a basis for further research. This chapter reviews the structure of the nervous system and theoretical models of pain.

## The Biomedical and Biopsychosocial Models

Two theoretical models influence our current thinking about the treatment of disease and tissue damage. The biomedical model is the oldest. Originating in ancient Greece and codified by Descartes in the seventeenth century, it assumes that an individual's complaints and symptoms are directly related to a specific disease state which can be confirmed by medical evaluation and tests of tissue damage and impairment. Appropriate medical intervention is then directed toward correcting the pathology. Referred to as a dualistic model, it conceptualizes the mind and body as separate entities. Symptoms originate either from the body (somatogenic) or from the mind (psychogenic). For centuries it was assumed that the cause of a patient's complaints was psychological in nature if medical evaluation did not identify physical pathology or if medical intervention failed to alleviate the patient's suffering. Even today, the cause of the continuation of physical complaint after traditional medical evaluation and intervention is sometimes attributed to the possibility of psychological variables alone when, in fact, that may not be the case.

Another way of thinking about disease and suffering has become increasingly accepted over the last couple of decades. Referred to as the biopsychosocial model, this broader view suggests that the mind and body are an integrated and dynamic system. The course of a disease or recovery from injury is determined by the interaction of physiological mechanisms, psychological factors, and sociocultural influences. Physical pathology alone does not always account for the course of an illness or the experience of suffering. This model has generated volumes of research and is becoming more influential in our approach to clinical treatment.

### How Does the Nervous System Work?

A review of the basic structure of the nervous system and how it operates will be helpful as we explore the complexity of the problem of pain and how different treatment interventions are proposed to work. Throughout the remainder of this book reference will be made to nerve pathways, neurotransmitters, and other nervous system components involved in the experience of pain.

The nervous system is a communication system. It is a complex combination of nerve cells that obtain information about what is going on inside and outside the body and then respond. The two major components of the nervous system are the central nervous system (CNS) and the peripheral nervous system (PNS) (fig. 2.1). The CNS consists of the brain and spinal cord. The PNS is composed of the autonomic nervous system (ANS) and somatic nervous system. Cranial nerves and spinal nerves are part of the PNS. The ANS is composed of the sympathetic and parasympathetic systems and controls all vital organ functions such as heart rate,

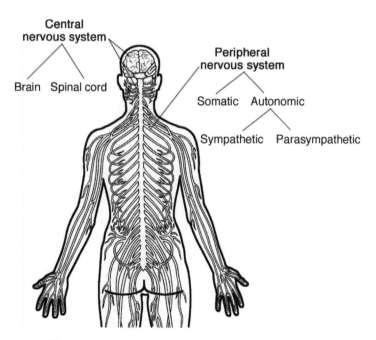

FIG. 2.1. The nervous system.

breathing, blood flow, digestion, workings of the bowel and bladder, and sexual functions. Information from the senses is transmitted to the CNS by the somatic system, which also carries information from the CNS to the muscles that move the skeleton.

### Neurons (nerves)

The fundamental units of the nervous system are special cells (neurons) that transmit signals to other nerves or other tissues (fig. 2.2). Like other cells, the neuron has (1) an outer membrane that acts like a screen, letting some substances enter the cell and blocking out others, (2) a cell body, or soma, (3) a nucleus, which carries genetic information that directs the cell's functioning, and (4) mitochondria, which generate cellular energy.

Unlike other cells, the neuron is a cord-like structure with fibers that extend from the cell body. These fibers are the axons and dendrites. Axons are the fibers that transmit signals

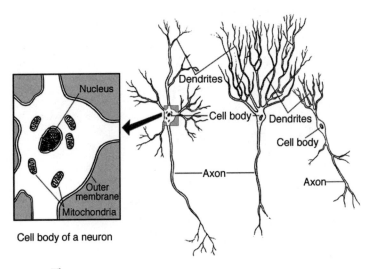

Cell body of a neuron

FIG. 2.2. The neuron.

away from the cell body, while dendrites transmit signals toward the cell body. Although a neuron generally has only one axon, it can have many dendrites. Messages are carried throughout the body by axon bundles called fiber tracts or pathways.

For messages to be sent from one nerve to another several things have to happen. A signal must be transmitted down the axon of one nerve and then cross over to the dendrite of another nerve. Neurons transmit messages by way of electrochemical impulses. Positive and negative ions (electrically charged particles) are distributed inside and outside the cell membrane. As stated, some ions are allowed to pass through the membrane and others are blocked. For example, water and carbon dioxide cross the membrane easily in either direction, but most other molecules cannot. Potassium and chloride ions cross less easily than water, sodium ions cross with still more difficulty, and some chemicals cannot cross at all.

Two competing forces, called the electrical gradient and concentration gradient, work toward achieving a balance in the electrical distribution of ions and the concentration of ions inside and outside the neuron. When the distribution of positively and negatively charged ions inside and outside the membrane is uneven, the membrane is said to be polarized. The inside of the membrane in all cells is slightly negative compared with the outside. Because ions with a positive charge are attracted to those with a negative charge, positively charged ions outside the membrane are driven toward the inside of the cell, such as positively charged potassium ions. When the concentration level of certain ions becomes greater inside the neuron they are then driven back toward the outside where the concentration is lower.

A neuron has a resting potential, which means that although the neuron is not transmitting (firing) a signal down its axon, it has stored electrical energy and is prepared to fire when the electrical potential reaches or exceeds a certain threshold. During a resting potential, the concentration of sodium is higher outside the membrane and it can cross the membrane only at a very slow rate. However, at threshold the sodium permeability increases, and sodium rushes across the membrane faster than it can be driven out. As the sodium concentration becomes higher inside the cell, a brief, massive electrical change in the distribution of ions occurs called an action potential. An action potential is sometimes referred to as an electrical or nerve impulse. When sodium ions enter the axon during an action potential, they passively diffuse to nearby areas, causing a change in the electrical potential at that point, and the sequence continues down the axon. Once the action potential gets started down the axon, it travels in only one direction and cannot pass back to the previously excited area. The movement of an action potential down an axon, the firing of the nerve, is called propagation of the action potential.

The action potential's rate of speed down an axon varies with the diameter of the axon and according to whether myelin is present. Some axons are covered with a myelinated sheath that is a coating composed largely of fat. The myelin sheath is interrupted at intervals by unmyelinated sections of axon called the nodes of Ranvier. An action potential cannot be propagated to the next segment of axon covered with myelin because the myelin serves as an electrical insulator and shield from sodium and other ions. Therefore, it jumps electrically to the next unmyelinated segment (node of Ranvier), and the normal type of propagation is used in this unmyelinated section. Action potentials travel faster down large, myelinated fibers and more slowly down small, unmyelinated fibers.

*Neurotransmitters*

To communicate with another nerve cell the signal must be transferred across a gap, called synapse, between nerves. This transfer is accomplished by a type of chemical called a

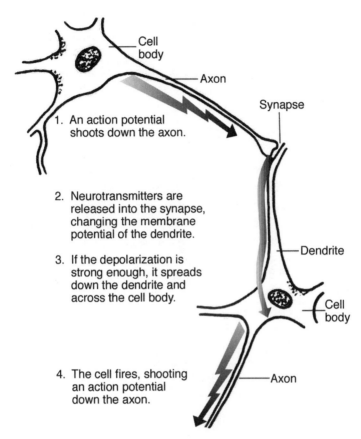

FIG. 2.3. Communication between nerves.

neurotransmitter released by the axon. The chemical spreads across the gap and triggers a change in the membrane of the receiving nerve (postsynaptic surface), creating an electrical signal (fig. 2.3). Whether the electrical signal is fired down the receiving nerve depends on the type of neurotransmitter released and what type of receptor it contacts. Receptors are specialized sites on the postsynaptic surface. The neurotransmitter is removed from the gap after it has interacted with its receptor. An enzyme is released that can break down the chemical or it can be transported back to the sending nerve (presynaptic surface), a process called reuptake. Over fifty known neurotransmitters affect our behaviors and mental processes. These include acetylcholine, norepinephrine, serotonin, and dopamine.

*Central Nervous System*

The brain is protected by the skull and controls our ability, among other things, to think, feel, move, and breathe. It is the body's master computer that receives and sends messages to and from all regions of the body. An extension of the brain is the spinal cord that extends from the base of the skull to the lower back. The spinal cord's main function is to relay messages throughout the body. It is protected by the spinal column, which is a bony structure composed of thirty-three vertebrae. The vertebrae are separated by disks. A disk is a spongy material that acts as a shock absorber, allowing our backs to move and bend. The vertebrae are held together by ligaments. The spinal column is divided into five sections: neck (cervical), upper back (thoracic), lower back (lumbar), back of pelvis (sacrum), and tailbone (coccyx) (fig. 2.4).

Thirty-one pairs of spinal nerves extend from the spinal cord to specific parts of the body. Although the spinal cord ends in the lumbar area of the spinal column at the level of the second lumbar vertebra, spinal nerves continue. This section is a tapering bundle of spinal nerves referred to as cauda equina because it resembles a horse's tail (fig. 2.5).

Information about muscle control and sensation is relayed to and from the brain by spinal nerves. Afferent nerves are those that transmit impulses from the periphery toward the central nervous system. Sensory information is relayed about a specific area of the skin to the brain from sensory areas called dermatomes (fig. 2.6). These areas contain nerve fibers or receptors from a single spinal root nerve. Messages from

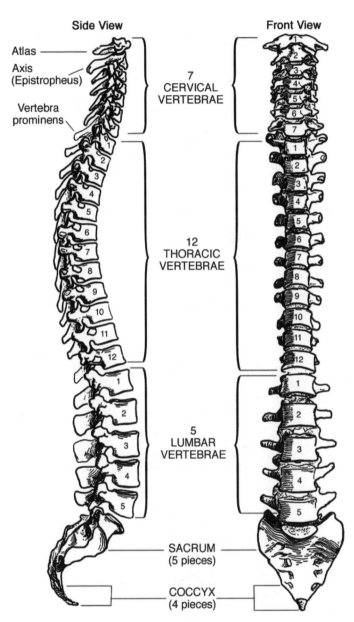

FIG. 2.4. The spinal column.

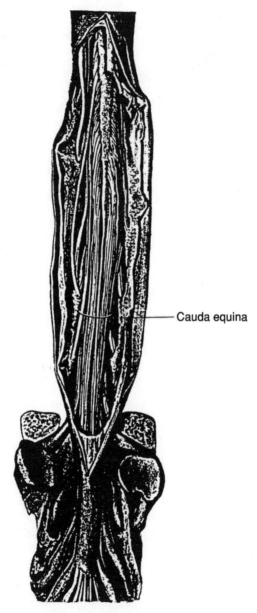

Cauda equina

FIG. 2.5. Cauda equina.

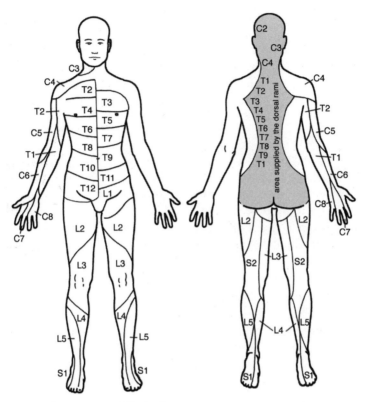

FIG. 2.6. Dermatomes of the body.

the central nervous system to the periphery are transmitted by efferent nerves.

The system is integrated, with certain nerve pathways of the spinal cord carrying sensory (temperature, pain, touch) information and other pathways transporting information about motor (movement) function. For example, if we touch something hot, the message "hot" travels from the hand through the nerve to the spinal cord. Once it reaches the spinal cord, two primary actions occur. A message is sent back through the nerve to our hand and we quickly move our hand away from the source of pain. This movement is called a reflex because the response to an incoming signal is directly "reflected" back out. The message is also sent to the brain. Once the brain perceives "hot," a message is then sent from the brain back down the spinal cord through the nerves to our hand. If the reflex response has not moved our hand, this second message causes us to pull away from the hot surface.

### Nociceptors

Most pain originates when nociceptors (specialized nerve endings) are activated. We have millions of nociceptors located in our skin, bones, joints, muscles, and internal organs. Some nociceptors react to several kinds of stimuli, and others are more selective. For example, some detect temperature and chemical stimuli, while others sense pressure and inflammation resulting from injury or disease. Certain nociceptors will respond to a pinprick, but not to heat.

When cells are damaged, they mediate pain and inflammation by releasing chemicals such as prostaglandins, potassium ions, serotonin, and histamines. Pain messages are then sent through the peripheral nervous system to the spinal cord and brain. Some pathways, containing A-Delta fibers, conduct signals faster than others containing C-fibers. The stimulation of A-Delta fibers results in sharp pain, while excitation of the C-fibers results in dull, burning pain. The transmission of pain signals can also activate the autonomic nervous system, which signals the release of hormones like epinephrine (adrenalin).

### Pain Theories

### Specificity Theory

Specificity theory proposes that a specific pain system sends messages from pain receptors in the skin along a specific pain pathway into the spinal cord and to a pain center in the brain. This model was first described by Descartes in 1664.

He suggested that the nervous system operates like a bell in a church bell tower. Someone pulls a rope at the bottom of the tower and the bell rings in the belfry. He wrote that a flame sets particles moving in the foot and the activity is sent up the leg and back into the head. In the head an alarm goes off. The individual then feels pain and responds to it.

The contemporary version of specificity theory is essentially that pain receptors in body tissue project by pain fibers and a pain pathway to a pain center in the brain. This traditional view of pain implies that the level of pain an individual experiences varies in accordance with the degree of actual tissue damage. The analogy of a telephone system suggests that if the wire carrying the message is cut, the transmission is interrupted or ultimately stopped. Therefore, a painful condition should be eliminated through appropriate treatment or surgical intervention. For example, if someone was suffering from back pain that was thought to be generated from a ruptured disk, repair or removal of that disk would cure the pain. Or, for nerve pain, the pain would theoretically be eliminated if that nerve were severed or ablated. Sometimes, surgeons actually amputated limbs in an attempt to eliminate the painful condition.

This theory was a major contribution. The physiological specialization of nerve receptors in the transmission of pain impulses is widely accepted, but the associated anatomical and psychological implications have not been supported through further research. Although the entire theory was given credence for many years, it falls short of explaining the phenomenon whereby individuals' responses to pain do not correspond to actual physical damage or disease or situations when pain persists beyond what is considered a normal period of healing. Someone can have a serious injury and not experience any pain if the person's attention is focused elsewhere. Researchers and clinicians have also observed that for individuals in chronic pain there is frequently little relationship between the amount of tissue damage and the

degree of pain complaint or physical disability observed.
Even when nerves sending signals to the brain are blocked
or severed, pain is not always relieved. For example, following
back surgery the individual often continues to experience pain
at the presurgical intensity level or even worse.

*Gate Control Theory*

In response to the many questions raised by the specificity
theory and other theories, Ronald Melzack and Patrick Wall,
then at the Massachusetts Institute of Technology, began a
collaborative relationship that led to the publication of the
gate control theory of pain in 1965. The gate theory differs
from earlier theories in several ways, but its main difference
is the concept of modulation. Incoming pain signals can be
inhibited and are not necessarily sent to the brain. Impulses
transmitted from pain receptors through the spinal cord to
the brain can be altered or blocked in the spinal cord, brain
stem, or cerebral cortex. Regardless of the type or intensity
of the noxious stimulus that causes the pain receptor to
become excited, the potential blocking ability of certain cells
along the transmission pathway can result in little or no pain
perception.

Essentially, this theory suggested that the substantia gelatinosa, which caps the grey matter of the dorsal horn in the
spinal cord, is the control center and governs whether pain
impulses are transmitted to the brain. The substantia gelatinosa is a unit of densely packed cells that extends the length
of the spinal cord. This site of control is referred to as the
"gate." Pain impulses can only pass through when the gate is
open or partially open, and not when it is closed. Substantia
gelatinosa cells are activated by large myelinated fibers (which
conduct nonpainful sensations) and inhibited by small fibers
(which conduct painful sensations). When activated, these
cells in turn inhibit large and small fibers from stimulating
T cells. T cells (lymphocytes) are specialized white blood

cells that have specific immune system functions depending on where they are located in the body. The stimulation of T cells in the spinal cord can trigger an action system that leads to the transmission of pain impulses and ultimately to the perception of pain in the brain. Some areas in the brain involved in the transmission or inhibition of pain signals include the raphe (descending pain inhibition), reticular formation (arousal/attention), brainstem (inhibitory area), thalamus (relay area), and somatosensory cortex (pain perception) (fig. 2.7).

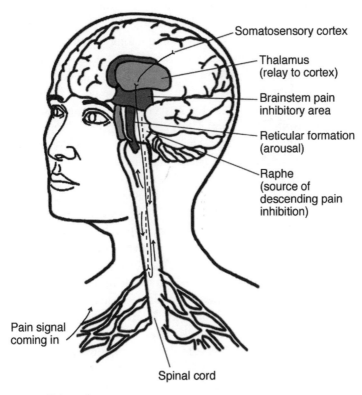

FIG. 2.7. Pain pathway.

The gate theory challenged the idea that pain is a simple sensation with a direct transmission line to a pain center. The concept of pain as a purely sensory (physiological) experience minimized the affective (emotional) and cognitive (thinking, perception) dimensions of the total pain experience. Typically, physiological and psychological aspects of pain were thought to be separate and totally different processes. The gate theory provided the conceptual framework for the integration of the sensory, affective, and cognitive dimensions of pain. It proposed a neurological basis for what was previously considered a purely psychological phenomenon. Our perceptions, thoughts, learning history, social relationships, and behaviors are thought to play a significant role in the pain experience.

The concept of a descending modulating system in which signals from the brain can open or close the gate to pain was considered revolutionary. Melzack and Wall proposed that other pain-inhibiting mechanisms involve the nerve fibers descending from portions of the reticular formation in the brain stem and from the thalamus and cerebral cortex (the central control system). The central control system consists of many neural areas in the thalamus and cerebral cortex and can be activated by stimulation of the dorsal horn transmission cells. Activation of the central control center triggers a descending blocking action. This action closes the gate to further incoming pain signals. The central control system in the cortex and thalamus affects attention, anxiety, anticipation, suggestion, and memory of past experiences. The cerebral processes were categorized as sensory-discriminatory, motivation-affect, and cognition activities. Sensory-discrimination gives information about time, location, and intensity. Motivation-affect indicates the presence of discomfort or unpleasantness, which triggers action to decrease noxious stimulation. Cognitive processes analyze past experiences, probable outcome, and the meaning of pain. The interaction of these processes influences pain perception and interpretation. The gate control theory is significant because it provides a possible explanation of psychological phenomena through the concept of a descending modulating system. Pain is a multidimensional experience. Our perception of pain and our reactions to it are influenced by the meaning we attribute to the pain-producing situation, our experiences or history, and our state of mind.

Although some problems exist with the physiological and anatomical aspects of this theory, it is widely accepted by scientists and clinicians. It has stimulated further pain research and has led the way to the development of multidisciplinary treatment interventions.

*Natural Pain Relievers.* How pain signals are blocked by the brain is not entirely clear. Two classes of substances seem to have a significant role in this descending system. The neurotransmitter serotonin is released by neurons descending from the brain. When the reuptake of this chemical is temporarily blocked, some individuals tend to experience pain relief. Serotonin is thought to play a role in the release of natural opiates called endorphins, enkephalins, and dynorphins that are painkillers our bodies produce. They act at many levels of the pain pathway, including the spinal cord, where they block the synapses of fibers that carry pain signals from the skin and other organs. These natural opiates also relieve pain when the adrenal and pituitary glands release them into the bloodstream as hormones.

Although we do not completely understand when and how the body eases its own pain, we do know that under certain physiological conditions this natural analgesic system is activated. For example, with certain types of physiological and psychological stress natural analgesic systems become activated. This may, in part, explain why individuals who are severely injured can perform lifesaving feats with no apparent pain. Also, research has shown that endorphins are released when individuals believe they are receiving a pain-reducing drug, even when they are given a placebo. Currently, there are pharmacological, behavioral, cognitive, and other interventions thought to affect serotonin levels and the release of natural opiates, as they are effective in rendering pain relief in some people. But even with all that we have learned, the challenge of finding a cure for chronic pain remains.

# 3. Seeking Relief

Those who know how close the connection is between the state
of mind of a man—his courage and hope, or lack of them—and
the state of immunity of his body will understand that the sudden
loss of hope and courage can have a deadly effect.

—Viktor E. Frankl, *Man's Search for Meaning*

## Who Treats Chronic Pain?

One of the most effective treatments for chronic pain is a
multidisciplinary approach that takes into consideration the
multifaceted nature of the condition. For optimal treatment,
regardless of the diagnosis, the psychological, social, and
physical factors involved in the chronic pain condition should
be addressed. This requires the coordination of evaluation
outcomes and treatment interventions among a number of
health care providers. For example, for back pain, health
care providers may include the family practitioner, surgeon,
physiatrist, anesthesiologist, physical therapist, psychologist,
and chiropractor. The treatment of chronic pain related to
cancer may include the family physician, oncologist, surgeon,
pain specialist, nurse, and mental health professional. With
a diagnosis of rheumatoid arthritis, the patient may receive
care from a rheumatologist, family physician, occupational
therapist, and others, depending on the course of the disease.
Coordination of care can become difficult when the patient,
frustrated and seeking immediate relief, begins to "shop
for a cure" with many physicians and collects a variety of
medications.

Multidisciplinary clinics are available for the treatment of many pain disorders in which assessment and treatment are provided through a coordinated treatment plan. However, more often, the health care professionals are not located within the same facility, and services are rendered at multiple locations. It is not unusual for providers to be located in different cities. At times this may become problematic, as communication and coordination of care among providers is necessary for effective treatment. Furthermore, effective management of a chronic pain condition depends upon the health care professionals sharing a common philosophy or understanding of the complexity of chronic pain. For example, the recognition of the importance of patients assuming an active role in their own care is vital. Patients should be considered members of their treatment team. Providing patients with information and education regarding chronic pain can help them to develop self-management skills.

Most physicians treat chronic pain, though they may not realize it or acknowledge it. Typically, family practitioners and general internists are on the front line in treating chronic pain conditions. These physicians usually serve as gatekeepers to specialty medicine. When we initially become ill or develop a pain problem, we usually seek help from our regular physician. After initial medical evaluation, a decision is made either to continue assessment and treatment or refer to a specialist. If the decision is to treat and that intervention fails, then referral to a specialist is more likely. In many cases family practice or internal medicine physicians continue to provide treatment, and medical care is coordinated with the specialist; or, after appropriate treatment has been rendered by the specialist, the patient is referred back to the regular physician for ongoing care.

The following discussion will define a number of medical and health care specialties that provide care to the patient with chronic pain. However, it should be noted that this list does not include every specialty and discipline involved in the treatment of pain. Further information can be obtained through some of the resources listed in the appendix.

## Anesthesiology

Anesthesiologists specializing in pain management are physicians who have received additional training in pain management after the completion of anesthesiology training. They serve as primary physicians or as consultants for patients experiencing problems with acute or chronic pain in both hospital and outpatient settings, and usually coordinate a multidisciplinary approach toward pain management for patients with pain.

## Cardiovascular Disease and Cardiology

Cardiologists are physicians who diagnose and treat diseases of the heart, lungs, and blood vessels. They can perform diagnostic and therapeutic procedures such as balloon angioplasty and cardiac catheterization. They may also oversee the medical care of patients requiring heart transplantation surgery.

## Chiropractic

Chiropractors are not physicians; they are trained to treat disease and injury by locating and adjusting a musculoskeletal area of the body that is functioning improperly. Emphasis is also placed on nutritional and exercise programs, wellness and lifestyle modifications for promoting physical and mental health.

## Counseling

Issues of spirituality and meaning frequently arise with patients suffering from a chronic disease process, terminal illness, and/or a chronic pain condition. Family members also may have related issues and difficulty coping. Many religions address these concerns and offer an important dimension in a multidisciplinary approach to pain management.

### Endocrinology and Metabolism

Some of the disorders treated by physicians with this specialization include diabetes, metabolic and nutritional disorders, and bone disorders such as osteoporosis. They also oversee the care of patients needing pancreas transplantation surgery.

### Family Practice

Family physicians are trained to prevent, diagnose, and treat a wide variety of ailments in patients of all ages. They are trained in areas which include surgery, psychiatry, obstetrics and gynecology, pediatrics, and geriatrics.

### Hematology and Oncology

This area of specialization includes physicians within a subspecialty of internal medicine who diagnose and treat disorders of the blood, spleen, and lymph glands, and all types of benign and malignant tumors.

### Internal Medicine

Physicians trained in internal medicine provide long-term, comprehensive care, managing both common illnesses and complex problems for individuals from the adolescent period throughout the lifespan. However, there are a number of subspecialty areas in internal medicine such as gastroenterology, geriatric medicine, cardiovascular disease and cardiology, endocrinology, hematology and oncology, infectious disease, and rheumatology.

## Neurological Surgery

Neurosurgeons provide services for the prevention, diagnosis, and medical and surgical treatment of disorders of the nervous system, and also rehabilitation. This may include the brain, spinal cord, skull, and associated blood supplies.

## Neurology

Physicians within this specialty diagnose and treat all disease or impaired function of the brain, spinal cord, peripheral nerves and muscles, and their blood supplies. These disorders include migraine, headache, Alzheimer's disease, Parkinson's disease, dementia, and other mental status problems.

## Nursing

Nurses are quite involved in the delivery of care to patients with chronic pain conditions and often function as part of a health care team in an inpatient or outpatient medical setting. They also are employed as case managers by insurance and rehabilitation companies to coordinate health care for patients among treating health care professionals.

## Occupational Therapy

Occupational therapists use directed activity and special skills in promoting and maintaining health, preventing disability, and rehabilitating persons whose normal growth and development have been interrupted by disease or injury.

## Orthopedic Surgery

This specialty includes the diagnosis and treatment of the extremities, spine, and associated structures. Physicians may utilize medical, surgical, or physical means to restore function, and may subspecialize in the orthopedic areas of hand surgery, joint replacement surgery, sports medicine, and others.

## Pain Specialist

Physicians can be certified as pain specialists by different boards. The criteria and requirements for certification differ depending on the board or organization. For example, the American Board of Anesthesiology (ABA) issues board certification in pain management after a physician has completed a fellowship training program in pain management approved by the Accreditation Council for Graduate Medical Education. Other boards do not require fellowships. Some of the organizations which offer board certification include the American Academy of Pain Medicine (AAPM), the American Academy of Pain Management (AAPM), and the American College of Pain Medicine (ACPM).

## Physiatry (Physical Medicine and Rehabilitation)

This branch of medicine emphasizes the prevention, diagnosis, and treatment of disorders, particularly those of the musculoskeletal, cardiovascular, and pulmonary systems, which may produce temporary or permanent impairment. The focus is to restore physical, psychological, social, and vocational function and alleviate pain.

## Physical Therapy

Physical therapists plan, organize, and administer treatment to restore functional mobility, relieve pain, and prevent or limit permanent disability for those suffering from a disabling injury or disease. Their patients may include individuals suffering from strokes, accidents, or permanent disability.

## Plastic and Reconstructive Surgery

Physicians in this specialty utilize surgical techniques to deal with the repair, reconstruction, or replacement of physical form and function involving the skin, face, hands, extremities, breasts, and external genitalia.

## Psychiatry

These physicians specialize in the prevention, diagnosis, and treatment of mental, addictive, and emotional disorders, including anxiety and depression.

## Psychology

A psychologist has completed a Ph.D. or Psy.D. in the field, and must hold a state license in order to practice. Regarding the psychosocial treatment of pain and other health care problems, psychologists generally have completed a residency or specialized training in the area of health or rehabilitation psychology. They address emotional, cognitive, behavioral, and interpersonal factors.

## Rheumatology

Rheumatologists treat connective tissue diseases which usually involve the joints, muscles, bones, and tendons. These disorders include rheumatoid and osteoarthritis, lupus, carpal tunnel syndrome, joint pain, and joint swelling.

## Surgery

General surgeons utilize a variety of surgical techniques to manage a range of conditions in almost any area of the body. There are many subspecialties within surgery, including vascular surgery, cardiothoracic surgery, transplantation surgery, and orthopedic surgery. Although surgeons generally provide pre- and postoperative care for their patients, ongoing care for the treatment of chronic pain following surgery is usually provided by the patient's regular physician or by health care providers involved in pain management and rehabilitation.

## Vocational Counseling

Vocational counselors facilitate patients' return to work by evaluating their physical and mental capabilities regarding job fit, and make recommendations regarding retraining and placement.

### Interdisciplinary Pain Programs

The term interdisciplinary, rather than multidisciplinary, is used to describe these programs because the health care providers share a common philosophy about chronic pain and actively communicate in the development and implementation of a comprehensive, integrated treatment program for the patient. Services are usually provided in one location. The treatment team generally consists of multispecialty physicians, physical therapists, occupational therapists, psychologists, nurses, case managers, and a number of other consulting specialties.

The International Association for the Study of Pain developed a classification of pain facilities which includes the following:

The *multidisciplinary pain center* is an organization of health care professionals and basic scientists who are involved in research, teaching, and patient care related to acute and chronic pain. Its wide array of health care professionals includes physicians, psychologists, nurses, physical therapists, occupational therapists, and other specialty health care providers. Multiple therapeutic modalities are available. These centers are usually affiliated with major health science institutions and provide evaluation and treatment.

The *multidisciplinary pain clinic* is a health care delivery facility staffed by physicians of different specialities and other health care providers who specialize in the diagnosis and management of patients with chronic pain. It differs from the multidisciplinary pain center in that it does not include research and teaching activities in its regular program.

The *pain clinic* is a health care facility that focuses on the diagnosis and management of patients with chronic pain. A pain clinic may specialize in specific diagnoses or pain related to a particular region of the body such as the head. This term is not used for a solo practitioner.

The *modality-oriented clinic* is a health care facility that offers a specific type of treatment *and* does not provide comprehensive assessment or management. Examples include nerve block clinics and biofeedback clinics. There is no emphasis on an integrated, comprehensive interdisciplinary approach.

### Evaluation of Chronic Pain

Chronic pain is a subjective experience and cannot be measured objectively with specific tests, at least not yet. Essentially, each health care provider assesses the impact pain has on different aspects of the patient's functioning. Assessment procedures typically differ depending on the discipline or medical specialty, the patient's relevant medical history, referring diagnosis, pain location and reported symptoms, level of dysfunction, and whether or not there is or has been an active disease process.

#### Medical

After performing an initial physical examination, a physician may order diagnostic tests to rule out the possibility of tissue damage or pathology. Some of these tests are general, and others are only performed within a particular medical specialty. For example, anesthesiologists may use spinal blocks and injections for diagnostic and prognostic purposes. Additionally important is a review of the patients' previous medical records and test results, as most patients with chronic pain have previously been evaluated and treated by other health care professionals.

*X-rays* reveal bone deformities or fractures. They are helpful in diagnosing certain diseases such as ankylosing spondylitis and osteoporosis, tuberculosis, and cancer. In the case of a ruptured disk, the disks themselves cannot be seen, but the vertebrae that appear too close together may indicate that the disk has ruptured or degenerated. X-rays are typically used to rule out certain conditions, and often their results help determine whether further diagnostic study is necessary.

*Computerized axial tomography (CAT scans)* are special x-rays, used with a computer to produce images of a specific area of anatomic tissue. They are used to evaluate the spinal cord and vertebrae and can help assess fractures, osteoarthritis damage, spinal stenosis (narrowed spinal canal), and tumors.

*Magnetic resonance imaging (MRI)* is used to assess muscles, cartilage, ligaments, tendons, and blood vessels. It can reveal whether a disk is protruding or ruptured. Additionally, MRI is used to look at possible infection. It uses a strong magnetic field and a computer to create highly detailed images of soft tissue.

*Myelograms* are used to provide a look at the spinal cord and spinal nerves. Before taking x-rays, the radiologist injects dye into the spinal canal. The dye, opaque to x-rays, outlines the spinal cord and nerves and can show a ruptured disk.

*Electromyogram (EMG)* is frequently used as an assessment tool in physical medicine and rehabilitation. It is a graphic recording of high voltage changes in a muscle. The EMG can show nerve and muscle damage and is useful in diagnosing the source of chronic pain involving the neck, back, and extremities.

*Nerve conduction studies* provide information about peripheral nerve function. They are used by neurologists to determine the presence and type of neuropathy and to localize nerve lesions and determine their severity. The nerve is stimulated electrically, and various factors are measured to determine the nerve's ability to carry the impulse.

*Diagnostic nerve blocks*, administered by anesthesiologists, can be an important part of the total evaluation of the patient's pain. They are used for diagnostic and prognostic purposes, and are useful in the evaluation of conditions such as pain mediated by the sympathetic nervous system. *Diskography* is a diagnostic procedure in which an x-ray "dye" is injected into an intervertebral disk of the spine and the disk is x-rayed.

*Physical Therapy*

The purpose of the physical therapy evaluation is to determine physical limitations in joint motion, muscle strength, and endurance. This initial assessment provides baseline measures which are used to establish treatment goals and measure the patient's progress. Self-report inventories to assess patients' perceptions of their pain and activity level are administered, along with performance and functional measures of physical ability. When assessing patients with chronic pain, the physical therapist takes into consideration motivational and cognitive factors which affect patients' physical capacity. For example, patients' fear of pain and reinjury and their perceived ability to perform a task can influence the evaluation.

*Occupational Therapy*

Occupational therapists evaluate and treat limitations in physical functioning. Physical strength and endurance are measured, along with an evaluation of the patient's ability to perform daily activities. Home and work-site evaluations are conducted to assess the individual's ability to function within those environments and the need for appropriate modifications.

*Psychology*

Psychologists conduct comprehensive assessments of the patient's emotional, cognitive, and behavioral status, along with taking a family, social, work and medical history. One purpose of the evaluation is to assess those factors known to affect treatment outcome so that a comprehensive treatment plan can be developed that is most beneficial to the patient.

*Pain intensity level.* An assessment technique used by all disciplines is the verbal measurement of pain in which patients are asked to quantify their pain on a 0-to-10-point scale. The health care provider simply states, "Rate your average or usual level of pain on a scale from 0 to 10 where 0 equals no pain and 10 is the worst pain you have ever had." Patients are sometimes asked to indicate their level of pain on a pain rating scale or visual analogue scale.

*Pain location.* The patient is asked where the pain is located or is asked to mark the areas of pain on a diagram of the body. The body diagram is also frequently used by physicians (fig. 3.1).

*Pain description.* The patient completes a self-report inventory that includes adjectives descriptive of pain complaints, such as "burning, tingling, sore, aching, radiating." This provides diagnostic and treatment information regarding the sensory, affective, and cognitive components of the pain experience.

*Frequency and duration.* Patients are asked when their pain is worse. How frequent is their worst pain and how long does it typically last? Is the pain constant? Does the pain vary in intensity? After pain has lingered for a long time, it is hard for some patients to quantify their pain or recognize any variability in pain intensity level.

*Factors affecting pain.* What factors decrease or increase the patient's pain? Patients often have difficulty specifying what influences their pain and will respond, "Everything I do makes me hurt." On the other hand, some patients target certain activities, positions, and behaviors that increase and decrease their pain. Patients who develop chronic pain following the diagnosis and treatment of carpal tunnel syndrome will complain of pain when lifting a coffee cup or cooking pan. Individuals with chronic neck or back pain report that

**Body Diagram**

Stabbing ---
Numbness ///

Aching   ***        Hot !!!
Pins and Needles +++

Cold (((
Tingling ===

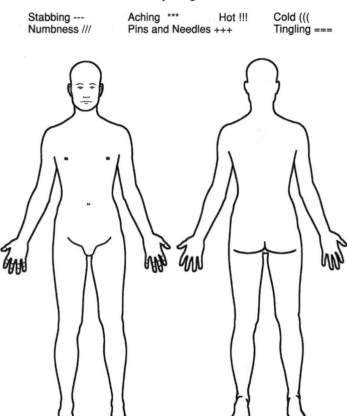

FIG. 3.1. Body diagram. The pain diagram is completed by the patient and is used as part of a comprehensive assessment to determine possible diagnosis and treatment interventions. Patients indicate the location(s) and type(s) of sensations they are experiencing.

their pain is increased by staying in one position too long or by sudden movements. Identifying factors that decrease their pain is equally difficult for some patients, who state, "Nothing gets rid of my pain" or "Only medication helps."

*Coping.* Cognitive, emotional, and behavioral responses to pain are assessed to determine how patients are coping with their pain and daily stressors. For example, patient perceptions and beliefs about pain are evaluated. If patients believe that all pain is disabling, they likely feel a sense of helplessness and an inability to control their pain. Their response to pain may be to withdraw from their activities.

*Activity level.* Information regarding work status and daily activities is gathered. How active is the patient during the day? How many hours does the person spend in resting or sitting to relieve pain?

*Self-report inventories.* Many of the above questions are included in a comprehensive assessment inventory that is completed either by the patient alone or with the psychologist. Additionally, questionnaires may be administered to assess the patient's emotional status (e.g., anxiety, depression), coping skills, perceptions, and other variables.

### Treatment Approaches

In the past, the management of severe disease and injury typically involved lengthy hospitalizations, bed rest, and extended periods of convalescence. This treatment approach was based on the biomedical or disease model which viewed patients as passive recipients of care. Today, our approach to the treatment of chronic pain emphasizes early recovery of function, and we address the role of psychosocial issues in our evaluation and treatment processes. Patients are now seen as active participants in their own care and part of a multidisciplinary pain management team. Multiple interventions are typically used to treat a chronic pain condition. Treatment regimens vary depending on the chronic pain disorder and symptoms and may target the cause of the pain or the pain itself. Interventions may include medications, nerve blocks and injections, physical or occupational therapy, rehabilitative exercise, electrical stimulation of muscles, implantable devices, cognitive and behavioral strategies (e.g., relaxation, biofeedback), and pain education.

## Psychological Approaches

Current research suggests that psychological and psychosocial variables are as influential, if not more so, regarding the individual's experience of pain and suffering as physiological factors are. The interaction of physical symptoms and psychological reactions to pain can develop into a "pain cycle" that leads to further dysfunction and suffering. Psychological issues may be addressed through use of a cognitive and behavioral treatment approach that emphasizes education, skills building, and self-management.

*Information and education.* Patients and their families are provided information about the differences between chronic and acute pain and specific information about their chronic pain condition. Important is the patient's understanding of factors that affect pain, appropriate treatment interventions, the patient's role in the management of pain, and the role of health care providers. Education emphasizes that most pain can be effectively managed. Misconceptions that serve as barriers to effective pain management are discussed. Education is provided through written materials and through individual and/or group therapy.

*Group therapy.* This type of therapy utilizes a psychoeducational model in which patients are provided with information about pain management and have an opportunity to interact in a supportive environment with other individuals who have similar conditions. A limited number of structured sessions are offered to assist patients in learning specific skills that will help them manage their pain more effectively. Emphasis is placed on the assumption of self-care responsibilities and quality-of-life issues. Helping patients feel that they have control over their pain and can participate in many activities they once enjoyed is an essential part of the group process. Cognitive/behavioral interventions such as stress management, problem solving, relaxation training, attention control/ distraction techniques, goal setting and self-monitoring are used. Additionally, patients' expectations, perceptions, and beliefs about chronic pain and related issues are addressed. Overall, emphasis is placed on the influence that cognitive (thoughts, perceptions, beliefs), affective (emotions), behavioral (what we do), and psychosocial factors have on chronic pain. Patients are helped to understand that the psychological, environmental, and physiological aspects of pain interact and influence each other. By combining and utilizing multiple interventions (e.g., exercise, relaxation, medication, coping statements), pain and suffering can be attenuated.

*Individual therapy.* Patients whose pain is particularly difficult to manage or who develop more severe symptoms of depression or anxiety may benefit from short-term psychotherapy. Again, the primary focus of treatment is to facilitate the development of self-management skills and help patients improve the quality of their lives.

*Cognitive-behavioral treatment.* The basic assumptions of the cognitive-behavioral treatment for chronic pain coincide with those of the gate control theory, which proposes that the experience of pain can be modulated by emotional reactions, thinking and perception, behaviors and environmental factors. For example, it has been demonstrated that intense emotional states and stress affect pain levels. When we become upset or angry (affect), we influence our physiological state. Our autonomic nervous system (see chapter 2) is activated, and we experience an increase in heart rate, blood pressure, and muscle tension. Muscle tension is also a factor that can cause an increase in pain.

Relaxation directly affects these autonomic nervous system responses, serving to close the gate to pain signals and thereby reduce painful sensations. On the other hand, physiological events can affect our emotional responses and our thinking. Changes in hormone levels and body chemistry can influence mood (affect). Furthermore, behavior (such as overdoing) can increase pain levels, and how we evaluate (cognitive) has an effect on pain levels. For example, an increase in pain may be seen as a sign of engaging in too much activity or as an indication that our condition is worsening (table 3.1). Research has shown that many of these interventions, particularly in combination, are successful in helping patients who suffer from conditions such as chronic headaches, cancer, rheumatological disorders, and back pain. Some of these approaches are discussed below.

**Cognitive reconceptualization** of the patients' pain and their ability to manage it is facilitated through a discussion of the gate control theory. Factors are identified that serve to open the gate or close the gate to pain signals being sent to the brain. This helps patients begin to alter their perceptions and realize that they have some control over their pain. For

**Table 3.1. Factors that tend to "open the gate" increase pain levels and factors that "close the gate" decrease pain levels.**

| Factors Affecting Pain | |
| --- | --- |
| *Open the Gate* | *Close the Gate* |
| Increased disease activity | Positive self-talk |
| Overdoing | Monitored exercise |
| Stress | Relaxation |
| Focusing on pain | Medication |
| Fatigue | Distraction |
| Improper body mechanics | Conditioning |
| Anxiety | Strengthening |
| Depression | Ice |
| Negative self-talk | Heat |

example, patients learn that with some painful conditions morning stiffness and pain are common. These symptoms do not mean that they have to remain in bed or necessarily limit their activities. By using stretching exercises, followed by a hot shower, they can possibly decrease their pain and stiffness. They begin to learn that there are interventions they can use, most often in combination, that allow them to have better control of their pain and function more effectively in their daily lives.

**Cognitive reappraisal** is a method whereby patients learn to monitor and evaluate their thoughts and replace them with more positive thoughts and images. Negative self-statements or self-talk tend to increase pain and suffering. When experiencing an exacerbation of pain and symptoms from overdoing, patients may respond by saying to themselves, "I can't do anything without causing my pain to be worse!" In reevaluating this statement patients may come to see that by pacing themselves and using other interventions, they can participate in many activities. A more rational self-statement or coping statement might be, "I did too much, so I'll have to pace myself more the next time."

**Problem solving** helps patients manage their pain by teaching them to use a systematic, objective approach to resolving issues. Problem-solving training may be viewed as helping individuals learn specific steps in identifying a variety of potentially effective responses to the problem situation, and it also increases the likelihood of selecting the most effective response from among these various alternatives. The goal of problem solving is to increase patients' feelings of self-control over their pain and develop more effective coping responses. Many patients continue to look to medicine for a "cure" for their pain and feel that, because it is a physical problem, they have no control over it. Additionally, some patients may feel that daily stressors (i.e., finances, work, family) are overwhelming and that they no longer have the coping resources to deal effectively with them. Patients are taught to specify a problem objectively and then identify alternative solutions. Each alternative is evaluated regarding its consequences so that the best one(s) can be selected. Patients also learn how to evaluate the effectiveness of the alternative(s) they choose to employ. For example, many chronic pain patients experience a sleep disturbance because of their pain. Problem solving is a useful tool in identifying possible solutions. Patients with back pain may identify alternative solutions such as changing their position, elevating their legs, eliminating daytime sleeping, sleeping on a firmer mattress, or using a relaxation technique.

**Attention control and distraction** are techniques that help patients learn to focus their attention away from pain or negative emotions accompanying pain. Attention to pain maintains or increases pain levels. Mental exercises such as counting, praying, and recalling lines of a poem are internal techniques that can be utilized. External distractions may include listening to music, watching television, reading or listening to another person read, talking to someone, playing a board game, or using the computer.

**Relaxation exercises** serve as attention control techniques and reduce muscle tension and other autonomic responses. There is some evidence to suggest that they also facilitate the release of endorphines, which are morphine-like substances that our bodies produce naturally. Breathing techniques, imagery exercises, and progressive muscle relaxation are used to induce a state of relaxation.

**Hypnosis and self-hypnosis** can significantly reduce some types of pain. Hypnosis is a state of highly focused attention during which alterations can occur in sensations, awareness, and perceptions. In regard to chronic pain, it is suggested that hypnosis is effective in changing the pain experience by shifting attention from bodily sensations. Relaxation procedures such as imagery and visualization are used. Hypnosis is generally used in the treatment of acute pain. In patients whose pain is long-term, self-hypnosis is more frequently recommended. Through skills training, imagery and hypnosis are taught to patients so that they can use these tools on their own.

### Therapies

Physical therapists, occupational therapists, chiropractors, and other professionals offer a variety of rehabilitative treatment interventions. Physical therapists, in particular, view activity, activity-related goal setting, and pacing of activity as integral parts of rehabilitation for patients with chronic pain. While many of the therapies discussed below are offered within specific disciplines, the general goals of rehabilitative therapy are similar across disciplines. Treatment plans are individualized and vary depending on the chronic pain condition, but the overall goals are to restore function, assist the patient in approximating normal activity, and decrease pain.

*Cryotherapy* is the application of cold to a local area. Possible benefits include analgesia, reduced inflammation, and decreased muscle spasm. Ice packs, commercially prepared chemical gel cold-producing packs, or towels soaked in ice water are typically used. Cold is usually applied for less than fifteen minutes. Ice is contraindicated for peripheral vascular disease, Raynaud's disease, connective tissue disease, or any condition in which vasoconstriction increases symptoms. Additionally, it should not be applied to tissue damaged by radiation.

*Thermotherapy* is the application of heat to a local area. Heat promotes sedation, muscle relaxation, and pain reduction. It induces vasodilation, which increases oxygen and nutrient delivery to damaged tissues. However, it is not recommended for use in patients with cancer because it can possibly stimulate the growth of cancer cells. Certain modalities, such as hot packs, are used to heat the superficial layers of tissue. Ultrasound therapy consists of sound waves and is used to heat deeper structures. Other methods include the use of hot packs, hot and moist compresses, electric heating pads, chemical gel packs, and immersion in hot water. *Electrical stimulation*, or electrotherapy, is the application of electrical currents to the body. Purported benefits include improvement of muscle contractility and endurance, decrease in spasticity, increase in range of motion, pain control, healing of tissue, and decrease in swelling. There are many types of electrical stimulation, but three of the ones used in pain control are high-voltage pulsed current (HVPC), or electrogalvanic stimulation (EGS); interferential current/medium current (IFC); and microamperage electric nerve stimulation (MENS). HVPC, or EGS, is a high-voltage wave form particularly effective in the treatment of open wounds. It is also utilized for reducing swelling and for the control of pain. IFC uses a medium current with special frequencies that allow the current to go deeper into the tissues for control of swelling and pain. The benefits of MENS are similar to those of HVPC and IFC, but it stimulates at a very low current level.

Transcutaneous electrical nerve stimulation (TENS) is most frequently used by patients for pain control. A small, portable device sends low voltage electrical current through electrodes placed on the skin. According to the gate control theory, TENS interferes with the pain cycle and closes the gate. TENS may also facilitate the production of endorphins, causing a reduction in pain perception. Many studies have shown that TENS is effective in reducing pain in some patients. For example, in a 1992 retrospective study, 59 percent of 1,582 patients with different pain etiologies stated that TENS use was successful in relieving or reducing pain.

*Massage* can aid in clinical evaluation by providing therapists information about muscle tone, localized muscle spasm, and nodules. In pain control it can be useful in softening and loosening scar tissue and producing relaxation.

*Traction*, or "unloading," is the technique of applying a pulling force produced manually or by a machine or device to part of the body to stretch soft tissues and separate joint surfaces or bone fragments. It can sometimes relieve pain caused by disk and joint problems, decrease muscle spasm, and aid in maintaining anatomic alignment.

*Manipulation* is a forceful movement performed by the therapist that stretches the tissue and helps restore range of motion. It differs from traction and stretching in that it involves a brief, quick maneuver. In some patients, it provides relief of pain and other symptoms.

*Exercise* is the cornerstone of treatment for chronic pain related to most musculoskeletal disorders. It is also helpful in the treatment of many other chronic pain conditions, as it strengthens muscles, increases endurance, and assists patients in returning to life activities. Exercise also mobilizes stiff joints, improves balance and coordination, and has positive effects on the cardiovascular system. Chronic pain patients have typically had long periods of inactivity, leading to decreased muscle strength and tightened joints which can cause an increase in pain. Depending on the chronic pain condition, graduated exercise regimens and home exercise programs performed regularly are quite effective in decreasing pain over time.

*Acupuncture* is derived from the words "acus," a sharp point, and "punctura," puncturing. It is one of the oldest forms of medical therapy and has been practiced in China for more than twenty-five hundred years. It consists of stimulating certain points on or near the surface of the body through insertion of needles. Acupuncture is thought to be similar to electrical stimulation, as it stimulates surface nerves as well as the nerves of deeper structures such as tendons and muscles. Much of the research on acupuncture is the result of uncontrolled clinical studies, but there is a body of information that supports the effects of it, especially when compared to narcotics and placebo. Some studies have shown that acupuncture increases the endorphin level in various parts of the central nervous system and affects neurotransmitters such as acetylcholine, norepinephrine, and dopamine.

*Nerve Blocks and Injections*

An injection is a method of forcing fluid into the body by means of a needle and syringe or a special device which uses compressed air. An injection may be intradermal, in which fluid is injected into the superficial skin layers; subcutaneous, injected into fatty tissue between the skin and underlying muscle; intramuscular, into a muscle; intravenous, into a vein; intra-arterial, into an artery; epidural, around the nerves of the spinal cord; intrathecal, under the membranes of the brain; or intra-articular, into a joint. Many different types of injections are given to decrease pain either by reducing inflammation and swelling or by blocking pain signals. These procedures are used for diagnostic, prognostic, and therapeutic purposes.

*Trigger point injections* are injections given to reduce soft tissue (e.g., muscle) aching and pain. Trigger points are specific points in muscles or soft tissue that cause pain (fig. 3.2). Injecting such points with a local anesthetic is effective in providing help for some patients that can range from a period of hours to permanent relief.

*Sacroiliac joint injections (SI injections)* are steroid injections that are given in the sacroiliac joints located in the lower back. The steroids reduce inflammation and swelling of tissue in the joint space and thereby reduce pain. A *facet joint injection* is the same type of injection, but it is administered in the facet joints located in the bony areas of the spinal column. Medications may include triamcinolone (Aristocort) or methylprednisolone (Depo-medrol).

*Stellate ganglion injection/blocks* are injections of anesthetic into sympathetic nerve tissue. These nerves are part of the sympathetic nervous system, which is part of the autonomic nervous system. They are located on either side of the voice box in the neck. The purpose of the injection is to block the sympathetic nerves. Patients may experience a reduction in pain, swelling, and sweating in affected areas of the

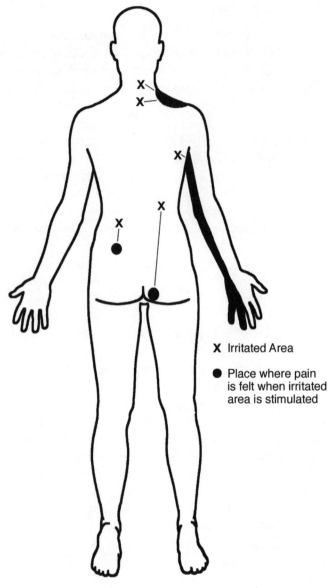

X Irritated Area

● Place where pain
is felt when irritated
area is stimulated

FIG. 3.2. Trigger points.

upper extremity. These blocks are helpful in the treatment of complex regional pain syndrome, sympathetically maintained pain, and herpes zoster (shingles) pain involving the upper extremity, head, or face. The lower extremity is treated with lumbar sympathetic blocks that are administered in sympathetic nerve tissue located on either side of the spine. Both stellate ganglion and lumbar sympathetic blocks consist of a local anesthetic. Epinephrine (adrenaline) or clonidine may be added to prolong the effects of the injection.

*Epidural steroid injections* are given in the epidural space, which is the area surrounding the spinal cord and the nerves coming out of it. Steroids work by reducing swelling and irritation in and around the nerves. A peripheral effect (outside the cell) is due to a reduction of inflammation or swelling. A central effect (inside the cell) may result from altering cell membranes and thereby decreasing neuronal excitability. The exact mechanism of action is unclear.

## Medications

Many different types of medications are used to treat chronic pain. Opiate analgesics and nonopiate analgesics are used to relieve pain. Antidepressants, anti-inflammatories, antiarrhythmics, and anticonvulsants are also prescribed. A medication regimen can consist of several different types of drugs which have different actions and are used in combination to treat the source of pain itself and to decrease the transmission or perception of pain.

*Nonopiate analgesics.* Nonprescription and prescription analgesics act on the nervous system and can temporarily reduce pain. Nonopiate medications, such as aspirin, suppress chemically induced peripheral pain, but do not block the transmission of pain. Aspirin and acetaminophen (Tylenol) are two common nonprescription pain relievers. Both are helpful in reducing mild to moderate pain. However, even with nonprescription medication, consultation with the physician is necessary if other medications are being taken or an individual is being treated for another health problem. These medicines can have a variety of side effects and can interact with prescription medications. The most common side effect of aspirin is stomach problems. Usually there are no side effects from the occasional use of acetaminophen, but excessive dosages or daily use over a prolonged period of time can cause liver or kidney damage.

*Opiate analgesics.* These drugs are prescribed by physicians for patients with moderate to severe pain. Opiates are derived from opium and include morphine, codeine, and other drugs that possess morphine-like properties. They act on receptors in the central and peripheral nervous systems and block the transmission of pain signals, altering pain perception. There are specific sites in the spinal cord and brain where morphine and similar drugs inhibit the transmission of pain signals. In the spinal cord, cells responsible for receiving and transmitting pain messages from the periphery to the brain are blocked. In the brain, opiates facilitate the transmission of messages down to the spinal cord that inhibit pain signals. It is likely that morphine and other morphine-like drugs produce analgesia primarily through interaction with mu receptors. These receptors are present in high concentration in the midbrain and the substantia gelatinosa of the spinal cord.

Many patients are fearful of becoming addicted to pain medications. However, addiction among patients who receive opiates for pain is less than 1 percent. A physical tolerance can develop if an opiate is taken over time, but this does not mean the patient is "addicted" or "drug-seeking." Additionally, the dosage or amount of medication one is taking does not suggest that one is addicted or is going to become addicted. Dosages vary depending on the age, weight, and type of pain the patient may have. If used as prescribed, opiates such as oxycodone (OxyContin Percocet), hydrocodone (Lortab, Vicodin), fentanyl (Duragesic Transdermal Patch), and morphine sulfate (Ms Contin) can be a safe and effective method of pain control for severe, intractable pain. An opiate-like drug also used in the treatment of pain is tramdol (Ultram). Common side effects include drowsiness, constipation, dry mouth, nausea, and vomiting.

*Anti-inflammatory drugs.* These medications reduce swelling and inflammation and thereby reduce pain caused by inflammation. NSAIDs (nonsteroidal anti-inflammatory drugs) can reduce inflammation after injury and in rheumatic conditions (e.g., arthritis, bursitis). Additionally, NSAIDs are used in controlling some types of cancer pain. Some of the drugs in this category are aspirin (Ecotrin), ibuprofen (Motrin, Advil, Nuprin), ketoprofen (Orudis), naproxen (Naprosyn, Anaprox), sulindac (Clinoril), meclofenamate (Meclomen), and piroxicam (Feldene). Common side effects include stomach upset and diarrhea.

NSAIDs reduce pain and inflammation by inhibiting prostaglandin synthesis. Prostaglandins are hormone-like substances that are produced by nearly all mammalian tissues via an enzyme called cyclo-oxygenase (COX), which comes in two forms, COX-1 and COX-2. Prostaglandins are derived from polyunsaturated fatty acids and mediate a wide range of physiological functions. In some tissues, prostaglandins serve a maintenance role, referred to as "housekeeping chores," and are turned on by COX-1, while in others they can cause inflammation and pain and are turned on by COX-2. Generally, NSAIDs are not selective in which prostaglandins they inhibit; they inhibit both COX-1 and COX-2. Although they reduce inflammation and pain due primarily to the inhibition of COX-1, they may also inhibit those prostaglandins involved in tissue maintenance, such as in the stomach lining, and thereby produce unwanted side effects. Relatively new, COX-2 inhibitors, which include Vioxx (rofecoxib) and Celebrex (celecoxib), are effective in reducing inflammation and pain without inhibiting COX-1, the enzyme that produces the essential prostaglandins. They reportedly lead to fewer gastrointestinal and other side effects that are common with the older anti-inflammatory drugs.

*Antiarrhythmics.* Antiarrhythmics change an irregular heartbeat to a normal rhythm by preventing or slowing abnormal electrical impulses in the heart. In a similar fashion, they reduce other abnormal electrical impulses along nerves. Antiarrhythmics lidocaine and mexiletine can relieve pain in many individuals with nerve pain. A loss of appetite and nausea are the most common side effects. Decreased alertness and drowsiness are also possible, particularly if an opiate is also being taken.

*Anticonvulsants.* Although normally used for seizure control, carbamazepine (Tegretol), gabapentin (Neurontin), valproate (Depakote), and topiramate (Topamax) can help some individuals obtain relief from nerve pain related to conditions such as diabetic neuropathy, trigeminal neuralgia, postherpetic neuropathy, poststroke pain, and migraine. They act to decrease abnormal nerve impulses in the nervous system by inhibiting norepinephrine uptake, stabilizing membranes, altering sodium, calcium, and potassium flux, or increasing the inhibitory activity of gamma-aminobutyric acid (GABA). Stomach upset, loss of appetite, and possible drowsiness are some of the common side effects.

*Antidepressants.* Imipramine (Tofranil), doxepin (Sinequan), amitriptyline (Elavil), desipramine (Norpramin), and nortriptyline (Pamelor, Aventyl) are tricyclic antidepressants (TCAs). In some patients this class of drugs has proven effective in reducing chronic pain, particularly in studies on nerve pain. TCAs have a sedating effect and can improve sleep. They block the reuptake of norepinephrine and serotonin that are known to be involved in the endorphin pain pathways at the central (descending) and spinal cord levels. Low serotonin levels have been found in both depressed and chronic pain patients.

Another class of antidepressants called selective serotonin reuptake inhibitors (SSRIs) have been found to be most effective in patients who are both depressed and have chronic pain. SSRIs include paroxetine (Paxil) and fluoxetine (Prozac). Other antidepressants often prescribed include venlafaxine (Effexor), nefazodone (Serzone), trazodone (Desyrel), citolopram (Celexa), bupropion (Wellbutrin), and mirtazapine (Remeron).

*Miscellaneous.* Muscle relaxants, antianxiety medications (e.g., Xanax, Klonopin), and antispasticity agents (Baclofen) are sometimes prescribed. Again, the class of drugs prescribed depends on the type of chronic pain disorder and the symptoms. Additionally, dosage depends on many factors, including individual pain tolerance levels.

*Implantable Devices*

Patients with severe, chronic pain who have not adequately responded to other treatments are sometimes considered candidates for the surgical implantation of pain-relieving devices. Before permanent placement, prognostic nerve blocks or trial placements are typically used to help determine the possible effectiveness of the device for the individual patient.

An intrathecal pump implant, sometimes called an infusion pump or spinal morphine pump, is a specialized device which delivers concentrated amounts of medication(s) into a spinal cord area through a small tubing (catheter). The type of medication(s) used depends on the chronic pain diagnosis. Opiates such as morphine, dilaudid, or fentanyl are infused for patients with cancer pain, failed back syndrome, and a sympathetically mediated pain. For disorders that involve muscle spasm, such as multiple sclerosis or spinal cord injury, antispasmodic medication (e.g., Baclofen) is used. This device is sometimes referred to as a Baclofen pump. Infusion pumps eliminate the need for oral medication and deliver medication

continuously. Placement of the pump is also an attempt to
eliminate or reduce breakthrough pain and other symptoms.
Another implantable device is the spinal cord stimulator,
or dorsal column stimulator. Low-voltage electrical impulses
stimulate nerves through small electrical wires placed on the
spinal cord. Nerve conduction, such as the transmission of
pain signals to the brain, is thereby interrupted. Stimulators
are usually considered for patients who have been diagnosed
with chronic, severe neuropathic pain and have obtained
minimal relief from other interventions. Neuropathic pain is
caused by damage to nerve tissue.

*Surgery*

Typically, surgery is performed to correct structural damage
or diseased tissue. Surgical intervention for relief of chronic
pain is generally considered a measure of last resort. Although, in some instances, surgery can provide immediate
relief from chronic pain, that relief may not be permanent.
Studies have shown that pain can return several months
following surgery, and its intensity may exceed presurgical
levels. Additionally, the surgery may destroy other sensations
and may cause a new source of pain. Physicians, therefore,
carefully weigh the necessity and benefits of surgery against
possible negative outcomes.

Operations to relieve pain generally involve severing con-
nections at major junctions in pain pathways or destroying
nerve fibers or parent cell bodies. For example, a sympathectomy is performed to relieve severe pain related to complex
regional pain syndrome or reflex sympathetic dystrophy. It
destroys certain nerves, called sympathetic nerves, in the
autonomic nervous system. Cordotomy is another surgical
procedure which severs nerve fibers on one or both sides of
the spinal cord. Besides surgery, other procedures used to
destroy tissue or nerves include the use of chemicals, heat, or
freezing treatments.

# 4. Taking Care of Yourself

We mourn the loss of ourselves—of earlier definitions that our images of ourselves depend upon. For the changes in our body redefine us. The events of our personal history redefine us. The ways that others perceive us redefine us. And, at several points in our lives we will have to relinquish a former self-image and move on.

—Judith Viorst, *Necessary Losses*

## Expectations

Most of us grow up with the idea that if we get sick or something happens to us, someone or something out there will "fix" us. Coming face to face with our own mortality is thought provoking and difficult to accept. However, the reality of having to live with pain day in and day out for the remainder of our lives can be even more disconcerting. Typically our expectations for the treatment of chronic pain are the same as our expectations for the alleviation of acute pain. We go to the doctor expecting a diagnosis and appropriate treatment that will restore us to our previous level of functioning. If there are complications, we return to the doctor expecting that, with appropriate intervention, the problem will be corrected.

Initially, when these expectations are not met, we often rationalize our situation by attributing a failure to find a cure to the incompetence of the physician or the inadequacy of the intervention. Consciously, or not, we reject the possibility that there is no cure for chronic pain. Because of our pain, we have lost much of our previous lives. We no longer enjoy participating in activities with our friends and families. We either have quit our jobs or struggle every day to maintain them in spite of the pain. In essence, we may feel that we are unable to participate in most activities that made our lives enjoyable. Conflicts may arise in our home because our partner becomes weary of carrying the responsibilities of the household and sometimes the financial burden for the family. Conflicts may also arise in our work environments because our coworkers feel we are no longer carrying our load. In desperation we continue our journey to find a cure for our pain and suffering and recover our lives. Our hope lies in knowing that somewhere there is a cure. Seeking treatment from many physicians is not unusual for patients with chronic pain conditions. Additionally, they may participate in therapies several times, take many different medications (often prescribed by different physicians), and turn to "alternative" medicine for answers.

As we approach the realization that there may not be a cure for chronic pain, we may become more and more discouraged and begin to lose hope. We may have heard from physicians or other health care providers, "There's nothing more that I can do for you. You're going to have to live with the pain." Our pain has now become "suffering," for we grieve the loss of our previous lives and, in part, have begun to lose that which we once knew to be self.

### The Emotional Impact of Chronic Pain

Any time we experience loss, we experience grief. Grief is defined as deep or intense sorrow or mourning which may include anguish, suffering, agony, distress, sadness, hurt, sorrow, unhappiness, torment, desolation, heartbreak, and helplessness. The greater the loss, the more emotionally intense the grieving process. Many patients with chronic pain feel they have lost almost everything important to them, particularly their physical health. In Elisabeth Kübler-Ross's book *On Death and Dying,* the process of grief is divided into stages which we may go through several times before coming to accept our loss. These stages include anger, bargaining, denial, depression, and finally acceptance.

The journey we embark on to find a cure is actually a grieving process which is colored by our expectations, perceptions, feelings, consequences, and others' reactions to us. We *deny* that there is no cure for chronic pain and continue to be solely dependent on the health care system for relief. We may *bargain,* anticipating that a cure will be forthcoming if we see one more physician or find someone who will perform a surgery. And, at some point, we begin to feel *anger* that may be directed at our health care providers for failing to render a cure or at our employer if the pain has resulted from a work-related injury. Often the anger is discharged toward the people who are closest to us, our family members. For those of us who are feeling a sense of helplessness, focusing on our physical limitations, undergoing frustration at not finding a cure, and dealing with the impact that pain has had on our lives, experiencing depression and anxiety is not unusual. Patients with low back pain show a major depression rate three to four times higher than the general population. Additionally, families of patients with chronic pain show a higher rate of depression.

The pain cycle involves factors that affect pain and are affected by pain. As stated, experiencing depression or anxiety is not unusual for patients because of their perception of their pain and the impact it has on their lives. In turn, depression and anxiety affect pain. It has been found that patients who are depressed experience higher levels of pain. Thus, our pain experience becomes a debilitating cycle in which pain and our emotional states interact to create more dysfunction and suffering.

## The Meaning of Pain

Our pain experience is influenced by our thinking. Our beliefs and perceptions of our situation can affect our reactions and coping responses to pain. For example, if we believe that any type of pain is a signal that something is wrong, we may continue to search for a cure and reject any other information or explanation for our condition and the management of it. Additionally, we may not understand that pain varies in intensity and that certain factors affect our pain levels. We may feel that we are unable to function with any amount of pain and that we are not "well" until the pain is totally gone. We may respond by trying to "wait the pain out," not understanding or accepting that it is unlikely to go away. Furthermore, we may perceive ourselves as powerless over our pain and without resources to deal with what is happening to our lives. In response, we may say to ourselves, "Everything I do causes more pain. Nothing takes my pain away. I can't stand this pain any longer." Feeling helpless, at times our thinking is characterized by overgeneralizations and catastrophic self-talk. These self-statements, along with our beliefs and perceptions, can have a negative impact on our pain experience and have been shown to worsen our condition.

## Behavioral Impact

Behavioral responses to pain include social withdrawal, decreased activity, overdoing, staying in bed, avoidance of activity, absenteeism from work, doctor shopping, taking medication(s) (sometimes inappropriately), and behaviors such as limping, facial grimacing, and verbal complaints of pain. Suddenly, we find ourselves spending most of our time

in activities that require no physical exertion or effort. We
may believe that when we have pain, rest is appropriate until
we get better. Family members and friends may reinforce
our behavioral responses to pain if they, too, believe that
all pain is disabling. They may encourage us to rest and
avoid any activity that may increase our pain. Or, on the
other hand, family members may respond with anger and
frustration because of our lack of participation in household
responsibilities and our decreased contribution to family
finances. These reactions can serve to increase our sense of
helplessness about our situation and cause us to think that
"no one understands or cares." In response to the pressure
of daily responsibilities, we may avoid activity and then try to
accomplish as much as possible in a short period which likely
serves to worsen our pain. The consequences of overdoing
serve to reinforce the idea that activity increases pain. As our
pain and depression become characterized by guilt, anxiety,
confusion, and hopelessness, we tend to withdraw even more
and to feel that we have few resources upon which we can
rely. Ironically, the focus of our lives becomes our pain, even
though it is the pain from which we are trying to escape.

**Breaking the Pain Cycle**

As we cycle back and forth through the stages of grief, we
struggle to find our way to accepting that we may have to
live with our pain. The journey is long and hard. We have
faced many barriers and followed many dead-end paths. Now,
with acceptance, we find ourselves willing to take a different
path—realizing that we may not find a cure, we seek a way
to take control of our pain and alter the negative effects
it has on our lives. It is at this point that we can begin to
move forward with our lives by taking an active role in our
own recovery. We can stop looking back to what we once
had and let go of some of the sorrow that we feel. We can

stop blaming others and ourselves for our pain and begin to assume responsibility for the management of it. Rather than seeing ourselves as a passive participant in our own care, we can begin to take an active role as the most important member of our treatment team. Reaching acceptance that there is no cure for chronic pain is not easy. It is a process, a journey.

### Seeking Answers

After we have been diagnosed with a chronic pain condition, the following steps may prove helpful.

#### Seek Medical Advice

Having confidence and good communication with our primary treating physician or pain specialist is a key to the successful management of pain. It is this physician who will oversee our treatment program, recommend interventions, make appropriate referrals, and answer any questions that we may have. Not all physicians receive training in the treatment of chronic pain conditions, so it is important that we find someone who understands chronic pain or who is willing to make a referral to a pain specialist or pain facility.

#### Make a List of Questions

Communication with the physician can be facilitated by making a list of questions before an appointment. Additionally, be prepared to indicate the location of the pain, its intensity, and how it feels (e.g., hot, burning, tingling). This assists physicians in their evaluation and subsequent recommendations.

#### Develop Realistic Expectations

We can expect to have some level of pain or a recurrence of pain throughout our lives. The physician will likely recommend several different interventions and may refer us to other health care providers or to a pain clinic, as one of the most effective treatment models for chronic pain is a multidisciplinary or multitreatment modality approach. Referral to a psychologist is not unusual and does not mean that the physician thinks the pain is not real. When referred to a mental health professional, many patients respond, "The pain isn't in my head!" Whether we are referred to a pain facility or to an individual practitioner, the likelihood is that a psychologist, psychiatrist, or other mental health professional will be part of the treatment team. Psychological and behavioral factors play an important role in the management of pain. It is unlikely that any one intervention will totally alleviate our pain, but we can expect that with the utilization of multiple interventions we can begin to learn to have some control over our pain and suffering.

### Set Realistic Goals

The primary treatment goal is to learn to manage our pain effectively and improve the quality of our lives. Measurable goals should be set so that we can evaluate our progress. Also, we should be realistic and establish goals that are attainable. For example, rather than someone saying, "I'm going to clean my house today," a more realistic goal might be to "clean my house this week by cleaning one room each day." Rather than a person stating, "I'm going to attend my daughter's tennis tournament," he or she might say, "I'm going to watch my daughter play her match tomorrow," which is likely a more attainable goal. Return to activity is gradual, and developing a plan to manage our pain is an important part of everything we do.

### Alter Beliefs about Pain

Many of our beliefs about pain may be inaccurate, and we should reevaluate those beliefs and make corrections as we gather more information. Chronic pain does not necessarily mean that we are disabled. It does not always require staying in bed. For most musculoskeletal problems resulting in chronic pain, one treatment is active physical therapy. In these and other chronic pain conditions, strengthening and conditioning exercises tend to decrease pain over time. Physical therapy and other behavioral interventions can help us begin to increase our activity level and find ways of participating in many activities that we once enjoyed. As the quality of our lives begins to improve and we begin to manage our pain more effectively, we will likely begin to feel better about ourselves. Increased activity and learning to manage our pain can decrease depression and anxiety.

### Seek Information

Health care providers are sources of information about chronic pain and appropriate treatment interventions. Ask questions. Additionally, relevant books are available and there is a wealth of information on the Internet. Many communities have chronic pain support groups. However, we must be selective when choosing a support group. Attend those that are proactive and take a problem-solving approach to managing pain. Too often support groups can become environments which serve to maintain our grieving process and do not offer paths toward recovery. Learn as much as possible about how to manage chronic pain.

### Comply with Treatment Recommendations

Compliance with treatment recommendations is quite difficult, particularly if we do not understand their importance or if they fail to bring immediate relief to our pain and suffering. For example, if we are prescribed an antidepressant for treatment of our pain and depression, it may take several weeks for the medication to become effective. Some individuals stop taking their medication or say that it is ineffective prematurely. Furthermore, home exercise programs can be quite effective in helping manage pain. When we first begin to exercise, particularly after having been inactive over a long period of time, we may experience soreness and muscle stiffness which we interpret as an increase in pain. Not understanding the importance of exercise and the symptoms we are experiencing, we may stop our home programs or drop out of a physical therapy program. Rather than altering our treatment program, discussing any problems or issues with our treating physician or health care provider is important.

*Assume Self-Care Responsibilities*

To effectively manage our pain we must be willing to assume self-care responsibilities. That is, after receiving education and information about how to manage pain, we must be willing to utilize and apply those skills in our everyday lives. Over time we can decrease our dependence on the health care system and begin to feel empowered by the skills we have learned.

We can learn how to identify factors that affect our pain intensity level and problem-solve when we have an increase in pain. By using several strategies we can exercise control over our pain and figure out how to participate in activities. For example, to attain the goal of attending our daughter's tennis match without experiencing a significant increase in pain, we should develop a pain management plan. With musculoskeletal pain, sitting in one position for a long period of time can increase pain, so it would be important to alter our position from sitting to standing occasionally. Sitting on a hard surface without back support, such as on a bleacher, can also contribute to pain. Taking a lawn chair or other chair that is comfortable and provides us support can help in managing the pain. Stretching our legs and arms occasionally can prevent stiffness. And, when we go home, a hot shower or bath may serve to relax our muscles. These sound like simple solutions to a complex problem, but when integrated into a plan, they can be quite effective.

Different types of interventions and different combinations of interventions work differently for different people. We must find those factors that help us manage our pain, and sometimes this is done by trial and error. Keeping a journal which includes pain ratings, coping responses, activity level, mood ratings, exercises, and medication intake can prove helpful in evaluating what works and in reporting our progress to health care professionals involved in the treatment. Additionally, as previously stated, compliance with medication regimens and other treatment recommendations is very important, and these strategies must be integrated into the pain management plan along with cognitive and behavioral strategies.

### Peace

A cure for our pain may not be available, but with a knowledgeable and compassionate health care treatment team, supportive family and friends, appropriate education, faith, and a willingness to be active participants in our own care, we can learn to lessen our suffering. We can find peace in our present and look toward tomorrow with hope.

# 5. Low Back Pain

Pain will force even the truthful to speak falsely.

—Publilius Syrus

Back pain, second only to the common cold as a leading
reason for visits to physicians' offices, is one of the most
significant health problems in the United States. In 1990 back
pain was listed among the most common reasons for hospital
admissions. The National Institutes of Health (Institute of
Neurological Disorders and Stroke) has reported that 70 to 85
percent of the adult population will experience back pain at
some time, with the annual incidence of back pain estimated
at between 15 and 45 percent. Symptoms are most common in
middle-aged adults, with no significant sex differences except
in pain secondary to disk disorders, which are more common
in men. Additionally, reported rates of low back pain are
generally higher for Caucasians than for African Americans
or other racial groups.

Approximately 2 percent of the work force sustain back
injuries each year. The total annual direct cost of treating
this group rose from $4.6 billion in 1977 to $11.4 billion in
1994. Approximately 25 percent or fewer of low back cases
are responsible for 75 percent or more of the cost. One study
reported that fewer than 20 percent of workers complaining
of back pain severe enough to seek medical intervention
continued to be off work after forty days. In California, 37.8
percent of all work-related compensation claims in a single
year were secondary to back injuries. Overall, it is estimated

that more than 50 percent of all compensation payments to disabled workers and health care providers is for back pain and related disorders.

Most patients with back pain recover quickly and without lasting effects on activity level or function. Typically, 60 to 70 percent recover by the end of six weeks and 80 to 90 percent by the end of twelve weeks. Further recovery is slow after twelve weeks. The recurrence rate of low back pain is quite high. One-year recurrence rates range from 20 to 44 percent, with lifetime recurrence rates of up to 85 percent.

Approximately two hundred thousand spinal surgeries are performed for back pain in the United States each year. From 1979 to 1987, rates of back surgery increased about 50 percent, while the rate of nonsurgical hospitalization decreased 33 percent. The increase of surgical rates was particularly high for fusions, which increased 100 percent from 1979 to 1990. Additionally, variations have been found in the rate of back surgeries in geographic regions and in other countries. For example, the rate of back surgery in the southern United States has been found to be twice as high as in the Northeast. In a study comparing the rate of back surgery in thirteen countries, the United States was found to have a 40 percent higher rate than all other countries surveyed (table 5.1). The increase in surgeries was affected by the development of new technologies and techniques, the advent of surgery as a subspecialty, and increased reimbursement by insurance companies and other third-party payors.

### Etiology (Cause)

The cause of low back pain is often difficult to determine. The majority of individuals with this complaint are diagnosed with nonspecific low back pain (NSLBP) rather than with a specific back pain disorder. NSLBP is defined as back pain complaints occurring without an identifiable cause. As medical science progresses, we may find the cause for low back

**Table 5.1. Estimated spinal surgeries.**

Estimated Rates of Spinal Surgeries

- Spinal surgeries estimated at 200,000 per year in U.S.
- 50% increase in rates of back surgery from 1979 to 1987
- 100% increase in rates of spinal fusions from 1979 to 1990
- Rates of back surgery vary in U.S. according to geographic region
- Rate of back surgery in southern U.S. twice as high as in the North
- Rates of back surgery vary among countries
- U.S. found to have 40% higher rate than 13 other countries surveyed

pain, but presently we are limited to conditions that include degenerative disk disease, herniated disk, spondylolisthesis, spinal stenosis, facet syndrome, spondyloarthropathies, systemic disease, and psychological problems. The diagnosis of sciatica is quite controversial as to its meaning and will not be discussed here. Fewer than 15 percent of back pains can be attributed to a specific cause.

*Degenerative Disk Disease*

Vertebral disks often degenerate as part of the aging process, with changes slowly occurring in surrounding area(s) as well. A narrowing of the intervertebral disk space usually occurs, and nociceptors in the outer anulus or dorsal root ganglion are stimulated and produce pain (fig. 5.1). Some people retain normal disk spaces throughout the aging process, while some

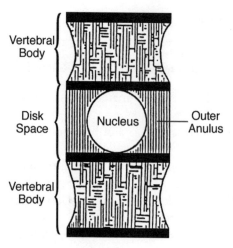

FIG. 5.1. Intervertebral disk.

experience gradual changes. However, not all individuals who have disk degeneration experience pain. We still do not clearly understand why some people experience pain and others do not. An episode of back pain can occur following a relatively minor trauma, such as stepping off a curb. Activities or other traumas may or may not produce symptoms.

Clinically, patients complain of chronic low back pain that is often accompanied by episodes of more intense symptoms. Pain is often felt in the buttocks, and nonspecific leg pain may be present. Pain is typically aggravated by activities that put pressure on the disk, such as sitting, prolonged standing, bending, or lifting. Common activities that may increase pain include sweeping, vacuuming, raking leaves, or mowing the lawn.

Degenerative disk problems usually resolve or improve within two to three days, no matter what treatment is prescribed. When the pain does not remit or recurs frequently, treatment programs consist of muscle strengthening and helping the individual learn how to use proper body mechanics, such as how to lift and how to get in and out of a seated position to avoid further trauma and increased pain. NSAIDs and other analgesics are frequently recommended. Epidural injections and blocks may provide short-term relief. In more severe cases back surgery may be considered.

### Herniated Disk

A herniated disk, also referred to as a protruding or ruptured disk, is one that has protruded through its surrounding structures (fig. 5.2). Pain can arise from nerve root compression or from pressure on the pain fibers in the supporting ligaments. Herniated disks are usually the result of injury, which may or may not involve lifting. Pain may occur immediately or develop over time. In many cases, patients cannot recall a precipitating event.

The amount and intensity of low back pain depends on the size and location of the herniation. For example, low back pain tends to dominate the clinical picture with a herniation that protrudes toward the spinal cord. Leg pain is more commonly the result of a lateral herniation that causes irritation or pressure on the corresponding lumbar nerve root. Pain usually increases with sitting, bending forward, and standing. Walking often relieves the pain.

The need for immediate surgery is quite rare. There is conflicting data about how much surgery helps to relieve pain over a long period of time. In some cases, conservative treatment has been shown to be as effective as surgery, if not more so, in attenuating pain and other symptoms. Only in the case of acute cauda equina syndrome is surgery considered absolutely necessary to avoid permanent nerve damage. Pressure on nerves in the cauda equina may cause weakness and paresthesias of the lower extremities, bladder dysfunction, and loss of muscle tone in the anus. Even if there is weakness, surgery may not be necessary if recovery occurs within several weeks. An aggressive conservative treatment program is

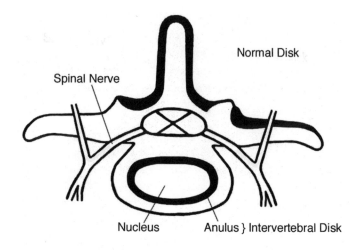

Normal Disk

Spinal Nerve

Nucleus    Anulus } Intervertebral Disk

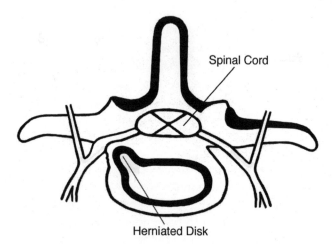

Spinal Cord

Herniated Disk

FIG. 5.2. Normal versus herniated disk. The disk material protrudes and can impinge or irritate the nerve.

typically established which includes physical therapy, medications, and, occasionally, spinal injections of steroids to reduce swelling. With conservative treatment most individuals improve considerably over six to twelve weeks.

## Spondylolisthesis

Spondylolisthesis is the forward displacement (slippage) of one vertebra (usually fourth or fifth lumbar) over a lower one (fig. 5.3). This condition can be easily diagnosed by x-ray, but we are not sure what causes the pain. It is thought that pain may arise from the disk at the level of displacement, the level above or below, or from secondary conditions such as spinal stenosis. Treatment depends on the grade of slippage or degree of ligament instability. For milder cases, back-strengthening exercises can achieve good results. Back support from a lumbosacral corset can also be helpful. More severe cases of instability may require surgical intervention to stop the slippage.

## Spinal Stenosis

Spinal stenosis is the narrowing of the vertebral canal. The incidence of this condition increases with age and most commonly involves the lower spine. With aging, there may be a gradual decrease in the space for spinal nerves because of a loss of disk height and changes in the surrounding ligaments. These changes lead to gradual encroachment of the nerve roots, usually occurring below lumbar vertebra 2 (L2). There is typically no involvment of the spinal cord itself, because the spinal cord stops at L2. Patients sometimes complain of deep, aching pain with a sensation of heaviness or numbness in the leg(s) radiating from the buttock to the foot. These symptoms typically worsen with walking. On the other hand, the distribution of pain depends on the nerve root(s) involved (fig. 5.4). Low back pain may be aggravated by specific body postures and/or physical exertion. Some patients may experience minimal pain while walking in a grocery store and leaning on the shopping cart and then have much greater pain when standing in the checkout line. Often there is minimal or no pain while a person is sitting or lying.

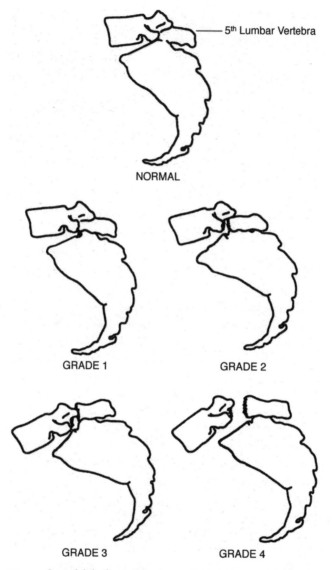

5th Lumbar Vertebra

NORMAL

GRADE 1

GRADE 2

GRADE 3

GRADE 4

FIG. 5.3. Spondylolisthesis. The forward displacement (slippage) of the vertebra can be progressive. Slippage is determined by x-ray and graded according to the amount of slippage with grade 4 signified by the vertebra's complete separation into two units.

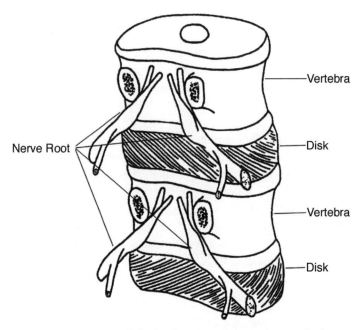

FIG. 5.4. Posterior view of the lumbar nerve roots in the vertebral canal.

Myelography with postmyelography CAT scans are often helpful in diagnosing this condition. Treatment varies according to the age of the patient, concomitant medical conditions, and the degree of pain and disability. Some patients stabilize without worsening. Other patients may benefit from epidural corticosteroid injections or blocks. In older patients with leg pain for whom surgical risk is considerable, spinal cord stimulation, such as TENS or an implantable device, has been effective. In patients who do not respond to conservative interventions, surgery is necessary, though risky.

### Facet Syndrome

Facet syndrome is back pain that is thought to originate from the side joints of the back. Facet joint pain is the primary problem in 15 to 20 percent of people with low back pain. However, there is controversy about whether facet syndrome is actually a distinct clinical entity. Diagnosis is usually made by injection with local anesthetic into the facet joint, which provides pain relief. X-ray is not helpful because radiologic appearance of the joints does not reflect the level of pain.

Patients typically complain of increased pain with prolonged standing and when changing positions from sitting to standing or lying to sitting. Usually, low back pain is experienced which radiates to the buttocks and upper legs. Treatment regimens consist of aggressive lumbar training to teach the patient strengthening exercises and proper body mechanics to use during activity. Additionally, short-term relief can be provided with facet joint injections.

### Spondyloarthropathies

This disease complex includes arthritic conditions such as ankylosing spondylitis, psoriatic arthritis, and sacroiliitis associated with inflammatory bowel disease. Back pain is produced by these disease processes and is usually more common in ankylosing spondylitis. A form of inflammation, ankylosing spondylitis can occur in many parts of the body but primarily affects the spine. Ankylosing spondylitis is more prevalent in men (197 cases per 100,000) than in women (73 cases per 100,000). Onset is typically between the ages of eighteen and twenty-five, with a range of fifteen to forty years.

The disease develops slowly over time. Low back pain or buttock pain is the first symptom in 65 percent of patients. Morning pain and stiffness are common, and fatigue may also be present. There may be pain and decreased range of motion in joints. Hip and shoulder joints may be involved. With advanced disease there may be decreased thoracic chest wall expansion. Interestingly, pain tends to increase with rest and decrease with activity. Medical history, physical examination,

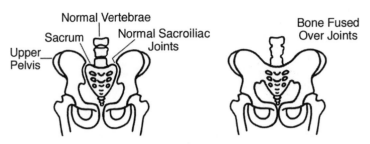

FIG. 5.5. Ankylosing spondylitis. Progressive changes in the joints of the lower spine and pelvis may result in fusion of the sacroiliac joints and vertebrae.

and laboratory tests are used to determine diagnosis. As the disease progresses, changes in joints, particularly in the pelvis, may be seen with x-ray, MRI, or CAT scan. In the early stages of the disease, alterations begin to occur in the sacrum and upper pelvis. As it advances, the sacroiliac joints become fused, and the joints between the vertebrae also grow together by bony changes (fig. 5.5). There is no cure for this disorder. Primary treatment is focused on relieving symptoms and improving spinal mobility if possible. Exercises designed to maintain mobility and posture of the joints are typically recommended. This condition may respond to some drug therapies used in the treatment of rheumatoid arthritis. Additionally, NSAIDs, physical therapy, exercise, and other forms of conservative therapy are all useful for pain relief and maintaining mobility.

### Systemic Disease

Approximately 5 to 10 percent of people with back pain have a systemic disease. Most often low back pain resulting from disease occurs in the elderly population. Except for compression fractures or osteopenia (any condition involving reduced bone mass) or cancer, medical causes for low back pain generally do not have a traumatic onset. The pain may initially increase with activity and diminish with rest. However, often the pain increases in intensity, becoming constant, and does not change with activity level. Additionally, whereas patients with low back pain may alter their position to relieve their pain, patients with systemic disease may not have a position of comfort.

### Psychological Problems

The interrelationship between psychologic factors and pain is well established. In some instances psychological and psychosocial factors precede the back problem, and in others the back pain itself leads to secondary psychological factors. In either case, most patients are believed to have some nociceptive input. However, the experience and expression of pain varies among individuals and at times may appear out of proportion to clinical findings. As an episode of acute back pain persists into a chronic state, psychological and psychosocial factors become more influential in the pain experience. Additionally, many patients with chronic low back pain suffer from depression and anxiety which can worsen their experience of pain and further diminish their ability to cope with their pain and the effects it has on their lives.

According to a publication by the International Association for the Study of Pain, the individual who reports pain or is observed to be suffering is not imagining pain. Malingering (the deliberate fabrication of symptoms) is rare. Chronic back pain is a problem that has biological, psychological, and social aspects, which must be addressed from the perspective of a biopsychosocial model rather than the traditional biomedical model.

### Assessment

### Medical History

The assessment of chronic or recurrent low back pain is quite similar to the evaluation of acute back pain. Acute low back problems are defined as activity intolerance due to lower back or back-related leg symptoms of less than three months' duration. As previously indicated, the majority of patients with acute low back problems spontaneously recover activity tolerance within one month. Most recurrent episodes of low back pain follow this same course. However, if the patient's pain has persisted beyond three months, then it is quite likely that other physicians have been consulted and previous treatments have been recommended. In this case, it is particularly important that the physician review previous medical records and any laboratory tests or imaging studies that were completed. This provides the practitioner with information which will be helpful in determining a diagnosis and prescribing appropriate treatments in a more cost-effective manner.

Initial assessment includes a medical history and physical examination. The medical history actually begins the treatment process, as it helps the physician establish rapport with the patient and build confidence. It also serves to direct the focus and evaluation of the physical examination; the physician gains information about influencing psychological and psychosocial variables, plans further diagnostic studies (e.g., referral for psychological/behavioral evaluation or imaging studies), initiates treatment, assesses progress and treatment outcome, and provides patient education. The medical history is an ongoing assessment tool which is used throughout treatment to help clarify symptoms and issues. Valuable information can often be obtained from family members and other interested parties.

Further assessment is completed to rule out the possibility of systemic disease or medical problems which may interfere with treatment or contribute to patients' pain. For example, a physical therapy program may be amended to accommodate patients with poor cardiovascular or pulmonary function. Degenerative arthritis of the hips or knees may cause patients to alter their walking, which could increase their back pain.

The onset, quality, intensity, and location of pain are also discussed. Knowledge of a particular event or trauma associated with the sudden onset of pain can assist the physician in determining the possible etiology of the pain. The physician may ask patients to describe the injury and what they were doing when it happened. For example, a patient who injured his or her back by lifting something heavy in a bent-over position may have herniated a disk. What happened and the position of the patient at the time of injury are important diagnostic variables. The quality of pain may include pain descriptors such as numbness, shooting, burning, aching, and tenderness. Burning pain may suggest neurologic or nerve pain. The location and distribution of the pain are also important, as different low back pain diagnoses have associated pain locations and patterns. For example, patients generally have secondary leg pain due to herniated disk. The quantification of pain or level of pain intensity helps the physician assess patients' perceptions of their pain and measure progress. Additionally, knowing the effects that different activities, postures, and positions (e.g., sitting or standing) have on pain levels assists the physician in arriving at a possible diagnosis. Other information gathered in the medical history includes psychological aspects of patients' pain (perceptions, mood, sleep), a work history, past medical history (including previous back injuries), and family history.

*Physical Examination*

During the physical examination the physician will evaluate the patient in different positions, such as standing, sitting, lying supine, and lying prone. Patients are usually asked if various positions or palpations are painful. Additionally, the physician assesses range of motion by asking patients to bend over and touch their toes while keeping the knees straight. They are also asked to bend backwards, keeping the knees and hips locked. Side bending is also assessed. As mentioned in previous chapters, patients with chronic pain play an important role in their own treatment process, which begins with the initial assessment. A clear report and presentation of symptoms by the patient can facilitate more accurate and timely diagnoses and aid in the development of an appropriate treatment plan.

Neurologic screening includes tests to determine possible evidence of nerve root impairment, peripheral neuropathy, or spinal cord dysfunction. These may involve testing for muscle strength, reflex testing, and sensory examination. Testing reflexes and having the patient perform certain movements such as squatting and rising, heel walking, and walking on the toes of both feet may provide evidence of specific disk and nerve root involvement (table 5.2). For example, positive reflex testing of the patellar tendon (knee) and observations of

**Table 5.2. Tests used to evaluate low back pain.**

| Neurological Testing for Lower Back | | | | |
|---|---|---|---|---|
| Disk | Nerve Root | Reflex | Sensation | Behavioral |
| L3-L4 | L4 | Patellar (knee) | medial leg, ankle, foot | squat and rise |
| L4-L5 | L5 | none | lateral leg and dorsum of foot | heel walking |
| L5-S1 | S1 | achilles | lateral foot | walking on toes |

STONEHILL COLLEGE

the patient squatting and rising may suggest the involvement of a lumbar disk (L3-L4) and nerve root (L4).

Occasionally, a patient with chronic low back pain will experience the onset of a secondary problem that may be overlooked. Such conditions as osteoporosis, resulting in a compression fracture, may be adding a secondary element to the underlying pain symptoms. Complications of procedures, such as an infection, or newly developing conditions, such as gout or kidney stones, may again be dismissed or overlooked in the patient with long-standing chronic low back pain. Suggestions of a new secondary problem may include a change in the description or location of the pain, or episodes of increased pain intensity.

*Symptom exaggeration and magnification* is not unusual for patients with low back pain that has persisted. Many health care professionals misinterpret this type of symptom presentation and consider it a sign of possible malingering. However, as earlier indicated, malingering is quite rare in chronic pain patients. There are usually other reasons for magnification of symptoms. The longer a patient experiences chronic pain, the more influential psychological and psychosocial factors become. If patients are not knowledgeable about their condition, they may be continuing to look for that "magic cure" and may be quite frustrated and disappointed in the medical treatment previously received. They may have seen many physicians and participated in physical therapy on more than one occasion. Additionally, they may not understand their role in the treatment process and the importance of assuming self-management responsibilities. They may not understand the difference between acute and chronic pain, and may still be looking to the physician to "fix" them. Exaggeration of symptoms may be a cry for help or the presentation of learned pain behaviors that have developed in response to a painful condition the patient does not understand.

## Treatment

Unless there is clear evidence of significant neurologic symptoms, such as nerve root damage, or of infection or tumor, the primary treatment for chronic low back pain is conservative intervention. Imaging techniques are not always accurate in determining the need for surgery. Degenerative changes in disks are found in pain-free adults. Progressive muscle weakness that significantly affects function is a strong indication for possible lumbar disk surgery. The cauda equina syndrome (loss of bowel or bladder control in a clinical setting with pelvic distribution of numbness) is a second indication for surgery.

Many patients with disk herniation are able to resume normal activity within one month of surgery. There is no evidence that delaying surgery for a period worsens outcomes. Approximately 80 percent of patients with surgical indications recover with or without surgery. Fewer than 40 percent of patients with unclear physiologic findings benefit from surgery. Evidence suggests that surgery may increase the need for future procedures. One study reported that 67.7 percent of patients treated with lumbar surgery for back pain reported that their pain was worse following surgery. Given the substantial number of patients with poor outcomes following surgery, use of prognostic indicators is crucial when surgery is being considered. Psychological and social indicators associated with poor prognosis can be identified with proper screening. Other factors considered include the presence of neurologic deficit appropriate to the involved nerve root, imaging evidence of compression of the involved nerve root, and positive straight leg raise (test suggestive of nerve compression).

A conservative treatment approach is most frequently recommended in the treatment of chronic low back pain and may involve referral to an interdisciplinary pain program that provides comprehensive care. Treatment focuses on providing education and skills training to patients with emphasis on the self-management of symptoms. Medical and psychological interventions, along with physical therapy, are typically prescribed. Treatments such as traction, TENS, epidural analgesics, and acupuncture are often helpful if used in conjunction with education and exercise programs.

The most commonly prescribed medications for patients with low back pain include the traditional nonsteroidal anti-inflammatory drugs (NSAIDs) and the apparently safer COX-2 inhibitors recently approved by the FDA. Muscle relaxants and antidepressants are also commonly used. Patients with complaints of stiffness appear to benefit the most from NSAIDs, because, given in higher doses, the drugs act to reduce inflammation. Otherwise, these medications function as analgesics and can often be used in lower doses or on occasion during episodes of increased pain. Patients with prominent muscle complaints appear to benefit from muscle relaxants such as cyclobenzaprine (Flexeril), methocarbamol (Robaxin), carisoprodol (Soma), and others. Additionally, seizure medications such as gabapentin (Neurontin) have been found to be effective in the treatment of spinal stenosis and other types of neuropathic pain.

Although clinicians have been reluctant to prescribe opiates in nonmalignant chronic pain, these agents may be quite useful in the treatment of specific back pain disorders. The risk of addiction is quite low. An effective dose should be prescribed, since ineffective dosing may prompt medication-seeking behavior. Long-acting opiates, such as OxyContin and Duragesic, may be practical and allow for return to more normal function and improved quality of life. However, in most cases, these drugs should be prescribed for a limited, defined period, with discussion (if not a signed contract) of the terms, potential benefits and risks, and obligations from the patient and physician. Overall, most medication treatment regimens provide only modest benefit and should not be viewed as the only treatment strategy, but should be incorporated into a multimodal intervention program. More aggressive treatment approaches, such as spinal stimulation, are sometimes indicated. Carefully selected patients may experience significant (greater than 50 percent) lessening of their pain. Administration of spinal opiates through a catheter allows some patients to obtain analgesia with fewer side effects than that achieved with systemic opiate dosing. These pumps require monthly follow-up, but the placement itself is generally safe if performed by an experienced clinician.

# 6. Nerve Pain

[W]e are not ourselves when nature, being oppressed, commands the mind to suffer with the body.

—William Shakespeare, *King Lear*

Neuropathy refers to a disease of the peripheral nerves, which carry signals throughout the body and connect the spinal cord to muscles, skin, blood vessels, and the internal organs. It is a disorder secondary to an insult to the peripheral nerves that can have a variety of causes. Approximately 20 million people in the United States suffer from peripheral neuropathy. Diabetes and alcoholism are the most common causes of this disease process in adults living in developed countries. Neuropathies associated with human immuno-deficiency virus (HIV) account for an increasing number of cases. In approximately 18 percent of cases a cause cannot be found. Common causes of peripheral neuropathy include metabolic disorders (e.g., diabetes, alcohol and nutritional deficiencies, hypothyroid), toxin-induced disorders (e.g., heavy metals, arsenic), infectious diseases (HIV, Lyme disease, posterpetic neuralgia), paraneoplastic disorders (e.g., lymphoma, multiple myeloma), immune-mediated disorders (e.g., vasculitis, Guillain-Barré syndrome), and hereditary sensorimotor neuropathies.

### Etiology

Peripheral neuropathy originates at the neuron (axon or cell body) or the myelin sheath. When the axon is primarily affected, it degenerates. Loss or abnormalities of the myelin can occur at multiple sites along an individual nerve. The majority of peripheral neuropathies can be classified into demyelinating, axonal, or a mixed pattern.

## Assessment

The assessment of peripheral neuropathies can be quite costly and time consuming. An in-depth medical history, including a family medical history, is completed to assist the physician in reaching an accurate determination regarding the cause of the neuropathy. Evaluation of medications is also important, as some can cause neuropathies. The diagnostic process may include nerve conduction and electromyogram studies, laboratory tests for possible nutritional deficiencies, MRI, and lumbar puncture. The progression of the disease is investigated and can point to a specific cause. For example, with trauma or ischemic infarction, the onset is acute, with more acute symptoms at onset. A chronic course over weeks or months is usually indicative of most toxic and metabolic neuropathies.

### Signs and Symptoms

The quality of pain, although variable, is usually described as burning, and most commonly affects the hands and feet. Symptoms of neuropathy depend on whether there is involvement of motor nerves, sensory nerves, or autonomic nerves. Involvement of motor nerves can lead to weakness, and some patients complain of having difficulty walking. Involvement of the sensory nerves can produce tingling, numbness, and pain, especially in the feet and hands. These sensory abnormalities are referred to as "stocking and glove dysesthesias." Autonomic nerve involvement can lead to changes in blood pressure and pulse, as well as gastrointestinal disturbances (e.g., diabetic gastroparesis).

The altered function of a nerve can occur with gradual injury, such as with chronic compression. Patients with compression neuropathies complain of a burning, tingling, and needle-like pain similar to that described by patients with acute nerve injury. In the gate control theory of pain, large diameter afferent fibers are thought to inhibit transmission of signals by the small diameter nociceptive fibers. Selective loss of large diameter fibers results in unopposed nociceptive signals and thus, pain. Hence, what in a normal person would not be transmitted as a painful sensation, such as light touch or pressure, is now perceived as pain. An example of compression neuropathy is carpal tunnel syndrome. This is an entrapment (pressure or squeezing) of a smaller peripheral nerve usually at the wrist, resulting in pain distributed along the first three fingers (fig. 6.1). Only later does a motor component become evident, with patients complaining of dropping objects and decreased ability to pinch.

Nerve entrapment can occur anywhere along the nerve fiber. Usually a narrowing of the canal that a nerve passes through will result in entrapment. At the wrist, this can occur in the setting of systemic diseases such as hypothyroidism, or with weight gain or pregnancy. Amyloidosis (a condition in which an insoluble protein is deposited in certain tissues), rheumatoid arthritis, and acromegaly (excess secretion of growth hormone) are among the associated conditions leading to nerve entrapment. The most common cause is repeated trauma, which can be minor. Patients may describe electric shock-like sensations in addition to radiating pain. Later, they may describe a deep aching sensation extending from the hand to the shoulder. Physical examination often demonstrates sensory loss in the distribution of the nerve.

### Treatment

Treatment intervention varies with the type of neuropathy present. However, in general, the management of neuropathic

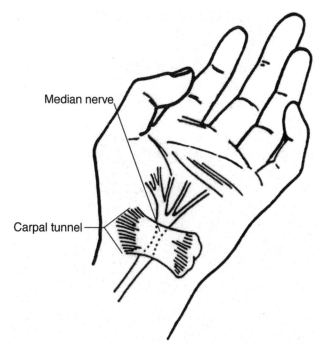

FIG. 6.I. Carpal tunnel.

pain involves the use of multiple treatments that include medication, psychological intervention, and treatment of the underlying cause of the peripheral neuropathy. For example, adequate blood sugar control in patients with diabetes can possibly delay the onset and slow the progression of the neuropathic process.

Many drugs have been tried as treatment for patients with neuropathies. Antidepressants are often prescribed first. These include tricyclic antidepressants such as amitryptiline (Elavil) and the newer SSRIs such as fluoxetine (Prozac) and paroxetine (Paxil). Although there are side effects such as dry mouth and cardiac arrhythmias to consider, tricyclic antidepressants appear to be more effective in relieving symptoms of neuropathic pain than SSRIs are. Tricyclics and SSRIs may help reduce pain because of their effect on the neurotransmitter serotonin (see chapter 2). Anticonvulsants such as gabapentin (Neurontin) and carbamazepine (Tegretol) are being used more frequently. Neuroleptics, antispasticity agents, and antiarrhythmics are helpful in some patients. Sometimes topical agents such as ethylchloride spray are useful. Capsaicin (Zostrix) and lidocaine are available as creams. Capsaicin (Zostrix) causes depletion of substance P, which may act as a neurotransmitter in this syndrome and affect pain. In cases of severe pain, opiates may be required. Some opiates are effective in blocking pain by stimulating endogenous opiate receptors affecting ascending pathways. In addition to these drugs, nerve blocks and injections also serve to relieve pain in some patients.

## Specific Conditions

There are many types of neuropathies, and most are quite complicated disease entities. The following discussions of postherpetic neuralgia, tic douloureux, diabetic peripheral neuropathy, and reflex sympathetic dystrophy are brief reviews intended to provide only basic information about these conditions.

### Postherpetic Neuralgia

Postherpetic neuralgia is a painful condition that may accompany or follow an episode of shingles. It is caused by the varicella-zoster virus, the same virus that causes chicken pox. Age is a major risk factor in the development of postherpetic neuralgia, with estimates of 50 percent for people older than fifty years and 75 percent for those above sixty-five years of age. Women are more commonly affected than men. In older patients, it often occurs in the ophthalmic division of the trigeminal nerve and can be severe. On the chest, it usually occurs along a rib, following the nerve under the rib on one

side of the body. The first symptoms are itching and a burning type of pain. These symptoms may be present for only a
few days or for several months before there is any evidence of
skin rash. The rash of shingles appears as vessicles or blisters
and may last for a few days or up to several weeks. This acute
phase when blisters are present should be treated aggressively
with antiretrovirals and, in some cases, corticosteroids, in an
effort to prevent the occurrence of a postherpetic neuralgia
type of pain that can be quite severe. If pain develops, it
follows the distribution of the peripheral nerves involved
in the area of the rash (see the discussion of dermatomes in
chapter 2).

The incidence of chronic pain with or following shingles
increases with advancing age, exceeding 50 percent in patients
older than seventy. Pain associated with postherpetic neuralgia
can become incapacitating and is described as stabbing,
shooting, steady, and burning. Patients may also experience
pain with light touch (allodynia). They often describe touch
or clothing against the skin as being painful. In some patients
over the age of fifty, or in the immunocompromised patient,
the pain may linger. Pain lasting more than one year occurs in
about a quarter of patients over fifty-five years of age and in
about half over seventy.

Pharmacological management of pain and related symptoms is very important. Drugs used to control postherpetic
pain include anticonvulsants and antidepressants. Capsaicin
cream (Zostrix) can be beneficial in controlling pain after
all skin lesions have completely resolved. It can not be used
around the eyes or mucous membranes, however. NSAIDs
and opiate drugs are sometimes required, as the pain may
become quite severe. Other interventions may include forms
of relaxation therapy and distraction techniques.

*Tic Douloureux*

Tic douloureux, also known as trigeminal neuralgia, is
a facial pain syndrome that usually develops in individuals

over fifty years of age. Classically described as knife-like or lancinating, this pain usually occurs unilaterally (one side) and more commonly affects the second or third branch of the trigeminal nerve. The trigeminal nerve is the chief sensory nerve of the face and the motor nerve of the muscles of chewing. It has three branches that are designated ophthalmic (first), maxillary (second), and mandibular (third). The cause is unknown, but in most cases the nerve is compressed by a blood vessel at the point of nerve root entry into the brainstem. In the majority of patients, however, the cause is unknown.

Patients describe small areas, sometimes inside the mouth, in which even light stimulation can trigger pain. Areas commonly involved are the eyebrow, the upper lip, and the lower molar teeth. Touch, cold, wind, and talking or chewing can precipitate painful attacks. The patient may experience pain-free periods for minutes to weeks, but long-term spontaneous remission is rare. Pain reportedly stops during sleep, but often recurs upon waking. Tic douloureux is not fatal, but it is one of the most painful afflictions known.

Anticonvulsant drugs such as Tegretol or Neurontin are used in treatment. Antidepressant medications also have significant pain-relieving effects in some patients. If medications are ineffective or produce significant side effects, neurosurgical procedures are sometimes recommended to relieve pressure on the nerve or to reduce nerve sensitivity. Other interventions found helpful include chiropractic adjustments, self-hypnosis, and meditation.

### Diabetic Neuropathy

Diabetic neuropathy is a nerve disorder caused by diabetes. Individuals can develop nerve problems within the first ten years after diagnosis of diabetes, and the risk of developing neuropathy increases the longer the patient has diabetes. About 60 percent of patients with diabetes have some form of neuropathy, but in many cases (30 to 40 percent) there are no symptoms. Approximately 30 percent of patients with diabetes have symptoms suggesting neuropathy, compared with 10 percent of individuals without diabetes. Diabetic neuropathy appears to be more common in patients who have had difficulty controlling their blood glucose levels and in patients over the age of forty.

The causes of diabetic neuropathy are unknown. High blood glucose levels cause chemical changes in nerves that impair the nerves' ability to send signals. Additionally, blood vessels that carry oxygen and nutrients to the nerves are also damaged. However, exactly how high blood glucose leads to nerve damage is unclear. Researchers are investigating several possible causes which include the effects of abnormal glucose metabolism on the amount of nitric oxide in nerves. Low levels of nitric oxide may lead to constriction of blood vessels supplying the nerve, contributing to nerve damage.

The symptoms of diabetic neuropathy depend on which nerves and what parts of the body are affected. Diabetes can result in the development of a number of neuropathies, with the most common type being peripheral neuropathy. In diabetic peripheral neuropathy the nerves of the limbs, especially the feet, are damaged. Common symptoms include numbness or insensitivity to pain or temperature and loss of balance and coordination. Additionally, patients usually experience tingling, burning, and prickling sensations. Patients may complain of sharp pain and extreme sensitivity to touch.

The primary treatment for diabetic peripheral neuropathy is prevention, aimed at delaying both the onset of symptoms and their progression. In a study conducted by the Diabetes Control and Complications Trial Research Group, intensive insulin therapy reduced the occurrence of neuropathy at five years by 69 percent compared with conventional therapy. In some cases lower blood sugar levels help reverse the pain or loss of sensation that neuropathy can cause. Drug therapy to reduce the pain and symptoms of peripheral neuropathy is implemented, along with an educational program that stresses the importance of insulin compliance and diet. Information is also provided regarding special care of the feet, which, because of loss of sensation, are prone to problems involving heat, cold, or skin puncture. Typically, a multidiscipline approach is most effective, given the multiple problems associated with this painful disorder.

### Reflex Sympathetic Dystrophy

Reflex sympathetic dystrophy (RSD), also called causalgia and complex regional pain syndrome (CRPS), is a chronic pain condition with sympathetic nervous system hyperactivity. Although RSD can affect most areas of the body, it frequently affects the upper and lower extremities. RSD is most commonly associated with minor soft tissue trauma or accident. For example, it can develop following placement of an intravenous needle, surgical procedure of the wrist or knee, fracture, or sprain. These patients experience immediate onset of severe pain, which is usually described as burning. Other symptoms may include hypersensitivity to touch, swelling, muscle spasms, skin changes, and joint tenderness. Vasoconstriction, leading to a cold sensation in the extremity, is accompanied by excessive sweating. Hair growth may be affected, and the extremity may appear mottled or splotchy. In severe cases, muscle wasting, chronic skin changes, periarticular osteopenia (bone thinning), and arthritis are present.

Although limited information is available on the incidence of RSD, this painful condition may affect millions. Some reports suggest that the syndrome occurs following 5 percent of all injuries. Although some mild cases resolve without treatment, others may progress through multiple stages and become chronic and debilitating. Treatment may include medication, nerve blocks, physical therapy, and psychological intervention. Physical therapy is a very important component of treatment, as atrophy of the muscles and decreased range of motion may occur in affected limbs. The goal is to keep the limb moving as much as the patient can tolerate to prevent further progression of the disorder. Providing patient and family education is particularly important, as patients typically display avoidance and resistance in moving the limb because of pain. Referral to a comprehensive, interdisciplinary pain management program that incorporates pain management skills training for patients is optimal. When medications fail to control the pain, sympathetic blockade may be tried. Transient relief may be achieved, but the duration varies. Initially, relief may only last hours to days. With repeated injections of drugs such as lidocane, longer periods of relief may be achieved and in some patients become permanent. In more severe cases placement of a spinal cord stimulator or a sympathectomy (interruption of the sympathetic nerve) may be considered. Surgery is a last resort.

# 7. Rheumatic Pain

The greatest revolution of our time is the knowledge that human beings, by changing the inner attitudes of their minds, can transform the outer aspects of their lives.

—William James

Recognition of rheumatic diseases dates back to prehistoric times. The term "rheuma," which means a watery discharge from a mucous membrane, was introduced in the first century. Rheumatic pain is associated with a variety of disorders characterized by inflammation, degeneration, and chemical changes in tissue structures, especially the joints and related structures, which include the cartilage, joint capsule, synovial membrane, bursa, ligaments, and tendons (fig. 7.1).

The musculoskeletal system consists of the bones and articulations of the skeleton and the ligaments, muscles, and tendons that connect them. There are over 150 painful and disabling musculoskeletal disorders. Many of these may be grouped under the umbrella of myofascial pain syndrome, but are sometimes referred to as myositis, fibromyalgia syndrome, fibrosis, fibromyalgia, myalgia, or myofascitis. Arthritis and other rheumatic conditions are the leading cause of disability in the United States, affecting 43 million persons in 1998, with a projected 60 million by 2020. In 1992 these conditions cost $65 billion in medical care and lost productivity, remaining among the leading causes of lost work time. One third of people disabled by rheumatic conditions are younger than forty-five years of age. Arthritis is an umbrella term used

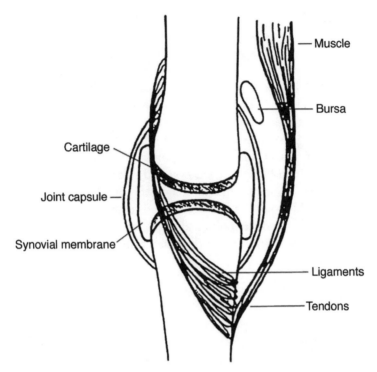

FIG. 7.1. Parts of a normal joint.

for various conditions of the joint structures. The two most common arthritic conditions are osteoarthritis and rheumatoid arthritis. Together these make up about 70 to 80 percent of arthritis cases.

### Myofascial Pain

Myofascial pain, sometimes called myofascitis or myofascial pain syndrome, refers to pain and inflammation in the "soft tissues" that include structures outside of the joint space, such as the bursa, cartilage, synovial membrane, and tendons, or muscles. It is usually caused by disease or injury to the muscle. The hallmark of myofascial pain syndrome is the "trigger point," characterized as a discrete painful area in the skeletal muscle. Trigger points often feel like a firm nodule or knot. Compression or pressure on these points can cause the sensation of referred pain in an area far from the original site. For example, shoulder pain may originate from a trigger point in the neck area.

The diagnosis of myofascial pain syndrome is established by demonstrating painful trigger points. These are consistent anatomically in both their location and referred pain pattern. There is no laboratory finding that is specific. Electromyographic (EMG) studies have also failed to show abnormalities. Thus, the most important diagnostic tool for evaluation and diagnosis still remains a thorough history and physical examination.

## Treatment

The goals of therapy in myofascial pain are to alleviate patients' pain and increase their ability to function normally. This condition is benign, and if treated aggressively can usually be managed effectively with positive treatment outcomes. Treatment approaches include education and psychological intervention, which help patients gain a better understanding of the condition, identify specific factors that affect pain, and develop effective coping strategies. Understanding the need for proper body mechanics, good work habits, and pacing in daily activities is important. Patients learn specific ways of managing stress and pain. Medications include injections of anesthetics, steroids, saline, or other agents into the trigger point to interrupt the pain cycle. Physical therapy modalities such as heat, ice, and ultrasound, as well as myofascial release (a form of deep massage) can give some temporary relief. These are typically used in conjunction with education, exercise, postural corrections, and training in body mechanics.

## Fibromyalgia

Fibromyalgia syndrome (FMS) consists of chronic, diffuse soft tissue pain with associated widespread discrete tender points. Patients complain of hurting all over for long periods of time, usually for years. FMS occurs primarily in women (10:1) and is usually experienced by people between twenty and sixty years of age. Approximately 75 percent of patients have associated fatigue, nonrestorative sleep, and widespread stiffness. Other common features include irritable bowel syndrome, abnormal sensations that may include burning or prickling, swelling, symptoms of anxiety or depression, and functional disability (an inability to carry out daily tasks necessary for normal living, such as bathing and dressing).

In 1990 the American College of Rheumatology adopted criteria for fibromyalgia. Before that time several terms had been used, including fibrositis. Because no evidence of inflammation ("itis") was present, this older term was dropped from use. The prevalence of fibromyalgia is estimated at 1 percent of the American population. Five percent of patients presenting to general internists and up to 20 percent of rheumatology clinic patients complain of some symptoms suggestive of fibromyalgia. The natural course of this condition appears to be a chronic pattern of varying symptoms and intensities, with periodic remissions. This common chronic pain syndrome will be a continuing source of medical and economic concern until the cause is better understood and more specific treatment approaches can be found.

Physical examination of a patient is notable only for its detection of the presence of tenderness. These tender areas frequently occur at muscle-tendon junctions, with palpation resulting in local pain only. There is usually no swelling or other signs of inflammation seen. Laboratory tests are used only to exclude other conditions that are also characterized by widespread pain and stiffness. Because fibromyalgia often occurs in the presence of other rheumatic disorders such as lupus or rheumatoid arthritis, specific tests may be ordered. EMG testing is typically normal. An electroencephalogram (EEG) non-rapid-eye-movement sleep anomaly has been found in some fibromyalgia patients, which may help explain chronic fatigue and diffuse aches. Many complain of not feeling rested after sleep. Subsequently, this may lead to inactivity causing aerobically unfit muscle that is then susceptible to pain with use.

Both fibromyalgia and myofascial pain syndrome are soft-tissue pain syndromes, but there are many characteristics that distinguish the two. Whether they represent two ends of the same spectrum is unclear.

### Treatment

Although the etiology of fibromyalgia is unknown, there are effective treatments that allow most patients to return to normal activity. Intervention includes limited medication, physical therapy, and education. Low-dose amitriptyline (Elavil) and cyclobenzaprine (Flexeril) may reduce the problems of sleep disturbance and decrease symptoms of fatigue. NSAIDs are often prescribed, but there is little evidence of benefit, and the usual side effects are common. Fibromyalgia symptoms are frequently intensified by emotional stress, and patients may experience depression and anxiety. Higher dosing of antidepressant medications and appropriate counseling may be required. Physical therapy focuses on muscle stretching, progressive strengthening exercises, and aerobic exercise. Myofascial release and cryotherapy may also be employed.

Clearly, an accurate diagnosis and explanation are essential ingredients for successful treatment. In more difficult cases, patients may not respond to simple reassurance, education, and physical exercise programs. Some patients complain that their lives are totally disrupted and resist involvement in appropriate treatments. In these cases the psychological aspects of this syndrome can have a prominent role in treatment outcome. Some patients benefit from cognitive and behavioral interventions that teach and emphasize symptom self-management and address the emotional components involved. In particular, these patients need to be reassured that their pain and associated symptoms are not related to an abnormality in the tissues themselves. As with other chronic pain conditions, changes can occur in the central pain pathways. Reassurances and explanations given to patients by their physicians can be helpful and possibly reduce fears and anxiety. The importance of active participation in exercise programs to promote better relaxation and hence better control of this amplified pain system is stressed.

Self-management of symptoms is a key in successful treatment of FMS symptoms and may be critical to functional outcomes. Teaching patients pain management skills may help them "push through the pain," especially in the first few weeks of physical therapy. Stretching and strengthening muscles is vital to a positive treatment outcome, as is stress and pain management such as relaxation, meditation, yoga, or similar activities. Patients are encouraged to select those interventions that work best for them and incorporate such practices into their daily lives.

## Osteoarthritis

Osteoarthritis (OA) is a degenerative disease that causes the breakdown of cartilage in joints, leading to joint pain and stiffness. Eventually, the surrounding bones are also affected. It is one of the oldest and most common of human diseases. Several other names are often used, such as degenerative joint disease, hypertrophic arthritis, or "old age arthritis." Osteoarthritis can affect any joint, but most commonly occurs in weight-bearing joints such as the knee, hip, or spine. It also affects the hand. Almost 21 million people in the United State have osteoarthritis. The risk of developing OA increases with

age, and the number of people with osteoarthritis will rise
dramatically as the general population lives longer.

Pain and stiffness are primary symptoms. Patients typically
experience increased pain with activity and relief of pain with
rest. Stiffness is often noted after periods of immobility (the
so-called "gelling" effect). Because of eventual changes to the
joint and the surrounding muscles, patients develop functional
impairments.

The economic impact of OA is enormous. Lost work days
are estimated at 2.5 days per month, and approximately 30
percent of OA patients are unemployed or retired because
of functional impairment. Costs remain high in part because of complications from treatment and the cost of joint
replacement.

Cartilage normally provides a smooth, gliding surface
for joint motion and acts as a cushion, or shock absorber,
between the bones. In OA the smooth surface softens and
becomes pitted. With time, large sections of this cartilage may
wear away, causing the bone surfaces to rub together ("bone
on bone"). As the cartilage breaks down, the joint may lose
its normal shape. The bone thickens, and cysts may form
near the joint. Bits of bone or cartilage may float loosely in
the joint space. All of these changes can create pain when
the joint is moved or used. In the knee, this may lead to a
"grating" or "catching" sensation. It becomes painful to walk
up or down stairs, and patients have difficulty getting up
from a seated position. Large muscles around the knee area
become weaker.

Bony growths (nodules) form in the fingers. In the end
joints of the fingers, they are called Heberden's nodes. If they
occur in the middle of the finger, they are called Bouchard's
nodes. Heberden's nodes appear most often in women and
sometimes occur early. They tend to run in families. In the
feet pain and tenderness occur most often at the base of the
big toe. Wearing tight shoes and high heels can make this
pain worse.

Factors involved in the development of osteoarthritis include genetics, obesity, injury, and repetitive overuse of certain joints. Some people are born with slight defects that make their joints fit incorrectly, as in the condition known as "bowlegs." Those with hyper mobile joints also have an increased likelihood of developing osteoarthritis. In some families OA may be the result of an inherited defective gene responsible for making a certain type of collagen, an important component of cartilage. This leads to early development of defective cartilage. Obesity increases the risk for OA of the knee. Changes in a joint (usually the knee) can also occur because of a sports injury, such as in football or soccer. Additionally, jobs that require repeated knee bending appear to increase the risk for OA of the knees. For instance, some miners and dockworkers have higher rates of osteoarthritis in the knees.

The diagnosis of osteoarthritis is usually based on the medical history and physical examination of the joints. Some other procedures such as x-rays may help confirm the diagnosis and determine how much damage has occurred. Occasionally, a procedure called arthrocentesis or joint aspiration is performed. Here fluid is taken out of the joint and lab tests are performed to confirm the diagnosis by excluding others.

*Treatment*

Treatment is usually aimed at both decreasing the pain and stiffness and improving joint function. This involves a combination of medications consisting either of Tylenol on a regular basis, of other pain medications, or of NSAIDs. Dosage of these may be adjusted based on symptoms and risks of side effects. Physical therapy, aerobic exercise, weight control, occupational therapy, and patient education are important additions to the treatment plan. Corticosteroids may be injected into the joint (intra-articular) following joint aspiration to relieve pain and swelling. Newer substances similar to normal joint fluid such as Hyalgan and Synvisc have recently gained increased use. Studies have demonstrated that use of these substances results in a decreased need for expensive and potentially dangerous oral medications. Topical analgesics in the form of creams, rubs, or sprays that are applied over the area of pain may provide temporary relief. Some serve as irritants that stimulate nerve endings in the skin and direct patients' attention away from the actual pain. Other preparations are compounded to include both pain medications and anti-inflammatory substances. Topical pain relievers containing capsaicin work by reducing the amount of substance P, a neurotransmitter.

Walking and water exercises do not stress the joints very much and are good for overall muscle tone and cardiovascular fitness. Weight loss is important for some, possibly in preventing the development of osteoarthritis of the knees, but certainly in reducing stress on the weight-bearing joints once arthritis has developed.

Surgery may be necessary when there is major joint damage and persistent pain. Osteotomy is one such procedure in which the bone deformity is cut and repositioned. Total joint arthroplasty (joint replacement) is another surgical option. The joint is replaced with metal, ceramic, or plastic parts. Researchers are currently seeking growth factors to drive the repair process so that damaged areas in the cartilage might heal and repair themselves, making surgical joint replacement unnecessary. Thus, these substances might allow the joint to remain in a reasonably functioning state for additional years.

## Rheumatoid Arthritis

Rheumatoid arthritis (RA) is an autoimmune disease that is characterized by inflammation of the joints, especially the lining tissues ("arth" means joint and "itis" means inflammation). It is associated with functional decline, frequent work disability, and premature mortality. RA occurs in approximately 3 percent of the U.S. population and is more common in women than in men (3:1). Many patients are young, but the incidence of RA is greatest among individuals aged forty to sixty years. It is estimated that up to 5 percent of patients are disabled to some extent five years after the onset of RA. Fifty percent are too disabled to work after ten years following onset. Considered a leading cause of disability, RA has an estimated economic impact of 9 billion dollars annually in the United States. It is an extremely disabling condition that significantly affects the quality of patients' lives and carries a high mortality rate.

In this disease, the synovium, or lining of the joints, thickens and may produce warmth, swelling, and pain in the joint(s). Commonly affected joints are the fingers, wrists, elbows, shoulders, knees, ankles, and toes. The linings of other areas of the body, such as the eye or lung, may also be affected. Joint involvement is usually multiple and symmetrical, affecting both sides of the body. One of the ways RA differs from osteoarthritis is in the pattern of joint involvement. For example, RA commonly affects the wrists, but usually not the joints that are closest to the nails, as in OA. Other joints that may be affected in RA, but rarely are in osteoarthritis, include the elbows, jaw, ankles, and shoulders. It is quite possible, especially as a person ages, to have both of these conditions.

A complete history and physical examination are primary in diagnosing RA. A history of symmetrical, multiple small-joint disease, with tenderness and swelling observed on physical examination, suggests disease. Certain laboratory tests such as the rheumatoid factor test are helpful only if positive. Many rheumatoid patients are anemic and have an elevated erythrocyte sedimentation rate (ESR), implying whole body inflammation and involvement. However, these tests (including the rheumatoid factor) are often normal or negative in early disease. Even in obvious cases of rheumatoid arthritis, 40 percent of adults will never have a positive lab test for rheumatoid factor. Thus, the fact that there is no single test that can establish or exclude this diagnosis may lead to delays in early diagnosis and treatment. Sometimes x-rays can be helpful, especially if the blood tests are not positive, but they may be more useful in following the progression of the disease and in evaluating treatment efficacy, since early x-rays may be fairly normal but later show joint and bone damage.

Almost all patients who have RA complain of joint pain and swelling. In some people the disease may be mild, with episodic "flares." In others, the disease is continuous and progressive over time, leading to tissue damage, joint deformity, and disability. Patients often feel sick, with decreased appetite, low-grade fever, anemia, and fatigue in addition to the painful joints. Descriptions of pain vary. Some patients complain of the worst pain with early development of swelling in their joints. This may be related to stretch fibers near the insertion site for tendons and ligaments. In later stages, pain may be related to chronic changes in the joints and surrounding tissues. Occasionally, pain may be severe even when the disease activity seems fairly well controlled.

About one-fifth of people with RA develop nodules (lumps of tissue) which are usually found just under the skin near joints or over bony areas but are occasionally elsewhere in the body such as in the lungs or eyes. Some patients develop inflammation of the lining of the heart or lungs. Dry eyes and mouth due to inflammatory changes in these tissues are also common (the so-called "sicca syndrome"). In rare instances, RA patients develop vasculitis (inflammation of the blood vessels) that can cause skin ulcerations and may affect internal organs.

## Treatment

As of yet, there is no cure for rheumatoid arthritis. Current treatments focus on relieving pain, reducing inflammation, slowing joint damage, and improving function and overall well-being. Drugs are the first line of treatment. Traditionally, medications used included NSAIDs and disease-modifying antirheumatic drugs (DMARDs) such as gold, azathioprine, or methotrexate. With the new COX-2 inhibitors, some patients may obtain a measure of relief from their pain and inflammation without experiencing the gastrointestinal and other side effects of earlier NSAIDs. The two currently available are celecoxib (Celebrex), approved for use in osteoarthritis and rheumatoid arthritis, and rofecoxib (Vioxx), which is approved for use in acute pain and osteoarthritis.

Analgesics are often used to help patients remain active and relieve pain. Steroids may be given, either into the joints directly or in small amounts by mouth on a daily basis during "flares," or when other drugs are not controlling the disease. The goal is to find the lowest effective dose that will not include many of the side effects of the steroids, such as bruising, weight gain, and bone thinning. Several new drugs for RA treatment have recently been developed and approved by the FDA. These are termed "biologicals" because they affect the immune system. Entanercept (Enbrel) and infliximab (Remicade) are two such drugs. These new agents have several advantages: they have a relatively quick onset of action (within two to four weeks), they bring about improvement in overall functioning, and, with continued use, they may actually prevent further joint damage. Others with slightly different actions may soon be available. Additionally, long-acting opiates have recently come into favor, primarily because of the safety profile of these drugs when used by patients taking other risky medications. If function improves without risk of damage to the joint structures, opiates may provide a practical approach to control of pain associated with rheumatoid arthritis. Adjustments in pain medications need to be made based on symptoms and the patient's needs, rather than by some predetermined formula, since there is great variability in patient complaints.

Exercise is important if the patient is to avoid declines in function but must not be overdone to the point of damage to the joints. Symptoms of overdoing may include increased pain and swelling. Physical therapists and occupational therapists may prove extremely helpful to rheumatoid patients. Water therapy can provide a method of exercise that does not increase joint swelling or pain. Rest can help, either during a general flare (the patient may stay in bed) or when a specific joint is targeted (for example, the patient may wear a wrist splint). Based on the disease activity in an individual at any given time, the amount of exercise, activity, and rest may vary. In some cases, joint surgery is necessary. This can range from a synovectomy (removal of the lining of the joint) to total joint arthroplasty (joint replacement).

# 8. Cancer Pain

Nothing I have learned in the past decade at the medical school seems to me more striking than the need of patients for re-assurance. . . . Illness is a terrifying experience. Something is happening that people don't know how to deal with. They are reaching out not just for medical help but for ways of thinking about catastrophic illness. They are reaching out for hope.

—Norman Cousins

More than eight hundred thousand cases of cancer are diagnosed each year, and pain is one of the most common symptoms. It is estimated that 30 to 50 percent of patients involved in active cancer treatment will experience significant pain. Approximately 50 percent of patients in intermediate or advanced stages of the disease suffer moderate to severe pain. Two-thirds of cancer patients will have pain that requires treatment.

During the early 1990s the undertreatment of cancer pain became a major public health issue. Several studies helped bring this matter to the forefront. One survey of more than twenty-five hundred patients revealed that over 50 percent did not obtain satisfactory pain relief. Another study suggested that between 50 to 80 percent of patients would not receive adequate pain treatment. These statistics were alarming, given estimates that in 90 percent of patients with cancer the pain should be controllable.

Only within the last couple of years have policies and programs been instituted requiring adequate treatment. The development of state cancer initiatives, release of pain management guidelines by the American Pain Society (APS), and the recommendation of specific policies by the Agency for Health Care Policy and Research (AHCPR) are among organized efforts underscoring the importance of providing aggressive, effective pain management to patients with cancer. The most notable progress to date is the recognition of pain as the "fifth vital sign." The Joint Commission on Accreditation of Hospital Organizations (JCAHO) is now requiring that pain assessment and treatment policies be instituted in all accredited hospitals and health care facilities. This establishes pain assessment as an important aspect of patient care, as is the evaluation of the other four vital signs (heart rate, blood pressure, temperature, and breathing rate).

Despite these changes and the availability of effective pain interventions, inadequately controlled cancer pain remains a significant problem. There are many factors that lead to undertreatment. For example, health care personnel may have deficient knowledge about pain assessment and treatment. Also, physicians and other health care personnel may under-evaluate the severity of pain and its interference in patients' lives. Underevaluation of pain is sometimes a result of poor communication between the patient and physician. Sometimes patients are reluctant to report the onset of more severe pain because of fear that the cancer is progressing. Additionally, the possibility of becoming addicted to medication is often a concern of patients and their families and can lead to stoicism (silent suffering) in patients.

Myths and misconceptions serve as barriers to improving the control of cancer pain and are often prevalent among health care providers, patients, family members, and the general public. Improvement in pain treatment requires that education be offered to all. The following is a list of educational points that are helpful in achieving effective treatment.

> 1. Patients will not always need increasing doses of pain medication, and they do not always become tolerant to the

medications prescribed. Additionally, increased dosages do not lead to addiction and other side effects in most cases.

2. Patients may become tolerant to the side effects of analgesics.
3. Pain relief sometimes involves the use of multiple drugs and coanalgesics.
4. Severe pain does not always call for the administration of intravenous or intramuscular drugs.
5. Addiction is not prevalent and is not a dangerous risk.
6. Cancer pain can be adequately relieved with drugs, and relief should always be attempted.
7. No ceiling dose exists above which opiates cannot be prescribed.
8. Not all patients on pain medications become physically dependent and experience withdrawal even with gradual tapering of the dose.
9. Pain medications should not always be prescribed on an as-needed basis.
10. Cancer pain can sometimes be managed effectively with analgesics.
11. Use of morphine or similar drugs to manage pain does not seriously repress respiration and shorten life.
12. Use of potent opiates to manage cancer pain does not imply "giving up" on the patient.

## Assessment and Treatment

People respond differently to the diagnosis and treatment of cancer, but it is usual for the patient and family to experience a range of emotions and behaviors during various stages of the illness. Beliefs, meanings, and expectations regarding diagnosis, treatment, possible treatment outcome, the role of health care providers, and the role of the patient and family influence coping responses. These responses vary over the course of the illness and may include fear, denial, anger, blaming, withdrawal, depression, anxiety, sadness, and hope. The patient may develop an intense fear in anticipation of possible pain and suffering. Health care personnel should work closely with the patient and family in helping them develop realistic expectations and an understanding of the treatment process. The relationship established between the patient and health care team is most important in the treatment of cancer and in providing effective pain management. Good communication can develop only if the patient feels a sense of trust and confidence in those who are rendering care.

Pain assessment should be ongoing throughout treatment, whether the patient is treated in a hospital or on an outpatient basis. Effective pain assessment involves determining what is causing the pain, evaluating pain characteristics (location, quality, intensity), and understanding the impact pain has on the patient's daily functioning and quality of life. Self-report inventories and pain intensity rating scales, in which the symptoms are rated by the patient, are frequently used, and methods of measuring pain that can aid in subsequent medical evaluations can be taught to patients and families. Health care personnel depend on the patient's self-report of pain to determine appropriate intervention. This point underscores the importance of the patient/doctor relationship and of maintaining open and honest communication.

Pain management should be discussed with the patient and family during the early stages of evaluation and treatment. Optimally, the goals of pain assessment and treatment are discussed through a mutual decision-making process, and a plan for ongoing pain assessment is instituted. This process can help reduce some of the patient's fears, clarify expectations, and define the roles of the patient and health care team. The goal of cancer pain management is to achieve a level of comfort that helps improve quality of life without compromising the patient's ability to think and function.

Acute pain may be accompanied by signs such as sweaty palms and increased heart rate, and may be related to procedures thought to be painful, such as bone marrow biopsy.

Increasing pain not associated with a procedure could signal the need for reevaluation of the cancer for spread and progression or for other underlying causes. The patient and family should be reassured that exacerbations in pain are not always an indication that the cancer is progressing, but may be related to another underlying condition or change in activity. Chronic cancer pain tends to be more complex. The continued presence of pain implies that total elimination may not be possible and that the patient needs some combination of relief and acceptance. In chronic pain, associated signs seen with acute pain such as fast heart rate, hypertension, and profuse perspiration are usually absent, thus providing no clues to the intensity of pain. Patients may appear "stoic" and may not exhibit many "pain behaviors" such as facial grimacing, verbal complaints, bracing, or holding the painful area. The absence of these symptoms should not lead either family members or the medical team to ignore or minimize the patient's distress.

Measurement of pain intensity is used in assessing the patient's progress and in decision making regarding appropriate medication intervention. The intensity of pain helps determine whether a nonopiate analgesic or a more potent opiate should be used. In many patients the pain has multiple causes, and the addition of other categories of drugs is often helpful. For example, the patient may develop visceral pain (coming from internal organs) or neuropathic pain. Additional drugs such as antidepressants, anticonvulsants, local anesthetics, and corticosteroids may be used. Breakthrough pain—intermittent worsening pain that is often related to a specific activity such as walking or eating—may occur and must be anticipated and addressed. This type of pain is best handled with supplemental analgesics that have a rapid onset of action and a short duration. Depending on the severity of pain, patient-controlled analgesia (PCA) that permits the patient to administer a preset amount of medication at preset intervals can be an effective alternative.

Some types of cancer pain are difficult to treat. With bone pain the mechanisms involved are unclear. Biochemical substances, such as prostaglandins, play an important role and most likely contribute to pain through an effect on peripheral nociceptors. Prostaglandins are released by damaged cells to aid in the healing process. Their actions can actually increase pain as a protective measure by causing swelling and inflammation at the affected area and by increasing the sensitivity of nociceptors to other chemicals that produce pain. However, with severe or ongoing tissue damage, the associated actions and pain become chronic and are no longer helpful. Prostaglandins are produced by an enzyme called cyclooxygenase (COX), and NSAID COX-1 and COX-2 drugs are prescribed to inhibit their release. The newer COX-2 inhibitors are reportedly safer for the gastrointestinal system and may be better tolerated with less nausea and esophageal irritation. Radiation may be successful in alleviating pain from metastases by shrinking tumor size. In patients with breast or prostate cancer, hormonal therapies are sometimes effective in reducing pain. For example, Lupron Depot, a member of a class of drugs known as gonadotropin releasing hormone (GnRH), works by inhibiting the production of the hormone testosterone, which may play a significant role in the growth of prostate cancer. Decreasing the levels of testosterone may also alleviate bone pain and some urinary problems associated with metastatic prostate cancer. Tumor invasion of bone may lead to compression fractures resulting in severe localized pain in the back. In some cases surgery may be required, particularly where there is spinal cord compression from a tumor.

Cancers associated with more severe pain also include pancreatic cancer and intracranial neoplasm. Pancreatic pain, characterized as a relentless, boring, and aching pain that often radiates from the abdomen into the thoracic back, may be relieved by assuming of a fetal position and made worse if patients lie on their backs. Intracranial neoplasm often

produces a severe, unrelenting headache and may precede
other neurological symptoms such as seizures, cranial nerve
weakness, muscle weakness, and lack of balance.
Unfortunately, the therapy itself may be a source of pain.
Treatment-related pain may cause confusion and lead to a
false assumption of worsening progression of the disease
itself. Painful polyneuropathy characterized by a burning
or tingling type of pain occurs with certain chemotherapy
agents. Radiation and chemotherapy may cause painful side
effects such as a sore mouth as soon as days and up to two
weeks following their use. This soreness may be severe and
can cause weight loss, dehydration, and weakness. Relief can
sometimes be obtained from the use of mouthwashes which
are composed of an anesthetic along with other ingredients.

The majority of patients will require analgesics, either
while they await responses to other therapies or to combat
side effects of therapies or for palliation of symptoms. The
oral route of administration of pain medications should be
maintained as long as possible to preserve the patient's inde-
pendence and mobility. Certainly the availability of oral agents
such as long-acting opiates (MS Contin, OxyContin) or transdermal fentanyl (Duragesic) has simplified this treatment. A
time-contingent schedule for analgesics that involves the use
of regularly scheduled doses is more effective than symptom-
administered analgesics given as needed. If analgesics are
withheld until pain is very severe, sympathetic nervous system
responses such as changes in heart and breathing rates and
increased nervousness may increase pain and make even
strong analgesics less effective.

Accompanying psychological factors such as depression
and anxiety may contribute to worsening pain symptoms.
Assessment and treatment by a psychologist or mental health
professional is often indicated. Educational and supportive
group sessions can assist patients in learning coping tools
that can serve to decrease anxiety and depression and give
them a better sense of control. Referral for individual therapy

should also be considered for patients with more severe depression and anxiety and if group therapies are unavailable. Instructing family members about cancer pain and involved emotional factors is also very important, as is providing them the opportunity to participate in support groups and family therapy.

Hospice care in the United States has been developed specifically to bridge institutional and home-based care for the patient expected to live less than six months. Care is based on quality-of-life issues and involves providing comfort to patients that is specific to their needs and wishes. A focus on pain and its relief is important throughout treatment, but is a special priority in patients with advanced disease who are dying. Hospice staff are trained to address the special needs of patients and family members at this stage of illness by offering compassionate caring, support, and intervention. Addressing the need for hospice services is usually difficult for the health care team because of what it signifies to the patient and family. Information about hospices should be integrated into education provided to the family throughout treatment, and specific recommendations for this service should be provided to the family early in the latter stages of the disease. Although it is a difficult situation, the patient and family can then begin to make informed decisions about the most effective alternatives for care.

In summary, the effective treatment of cancer pain requires an interdisciplinary treatment approach in which the patient and family members are seen as part of the treatment team. Primary care physicians, oncologists, anesthesiologists (pain specialists), physical therapists, occupational therapists, psychologists, pastoral counselors, nurses, and social workers are but a few of the health care providers who may be involved. Education, communication, coordination of efforts, and compassionate care giving are the cornerstones of effective cancer pain management.

# 9. Other Chronic Pain Conditions

English, which can express the thoughts of Hamlet and the tragedy of Lear, has no words for the shiver or the headache. . . . The merest schoolgirl when she falls in love has Shakespeare or Keats to speak her mind for her, but let a sufferer try to describe a pain in his head to a doctor and language at once runs dry.

—Virginia Woolf

## Interstitial Cystitis

Interstitial cystitis (IC) is a condition characterized by urinary frequency, urgency, and pain that is often excruciating. Onset is typically in youth or middle age, and 90 percent of the patients are women. This condition remains one of medicine's imposing clinical challenges. It is often associated with fibromyalgia and irritable bowel syndrome. An estimated five hundred thousand cases exist in the United States. Interstitial cystitis is often misdiagnosed, with the average time from onset of symptoms to diagnosis being seven years. Although previously thought to be primarily a psychiatric illness, it is a disease characterized by anatomic and physiologic changes within the bladder. However, the search for a cause continues, while intervention is focused on the treatment of symptoms.

The pain associated with interstitial cystitis is described by most as burning in the bladder, lower abdomen, pelvis, vagina, and pubic area. Pain increases with bladder filling and is relieved by bladder emptying. Menstruation aggravates the symptoms, and many women feel their symptoms worsen with sexual intercourse. Associated chronic sleep loss from frequent urination produces secondary psychological problems, such as depression. Making the diagnosis of IC requires a thorough history and physical examination. A cystoscopy under anesthesia with hydrodistention is usually performed. In this procedure the patient's bladder is filled with water so the physician can look at the bladder structure through a small lighted tube. The findings of a pale lining and shallow ulcers support the diagnosis. Small hemorrhages, which appear as tiny red spots, are common in the nonulcerative form. Later, a fibrous, contracted bladder may be seen.

*Treatment*

Once the diagnosis is confirmed, different treatment options may be discussed. Treatment usually begins with inhibition or control of histamine release through the use of antihistamines such as Atarax. NSAIDs may relieve symptoms in some patients. Treatments approved by the FDA have included instillation substances, such as dimethyl sulfoxide (DMSO), into the bladder. DMSO is a chemical that is believed to inhibit free-radical production, thus reducing pain and inflammation. Hydroxyl radicals (OH), which are free radicals (oxidants), are highly injurious to cells. DMSO substitutes for water in cells and neutralizes oxidants. DMSO can carry other substances across membranes and can be mixed with steroids, heparin, and anesthetics. Other measures such as alcohol instillation and steroids have been tried, but prolonged improvement has not been documented for these. Drastic measures such as removing the bladder have occasionally been performed, but unfortunately some of these patients continue to have their pain. These patients share many common features of reflex sympathetic dystrophy.

Recently, gabapentin (Neurontin) and pentosan (Elmiron) have been shown to be effective without excessive adverse effects. How these drugs act to relieve symptoms is unknown. Elmiron is the only oral therapy currently approved by the FDA for use in interstitial cystitis. Both Neurontin and Elmiron may provide a safe alternative to narcotics, since this pain is often resistant to opiates. However, Elmiron may lead to reversible hair loss, and it may take several months to control this condition.

Many patients with interstitial cystitis have an associated depression, so tricyclic antidepressants such as amitriptyline (Elavil) and doxepin (Sinequan) provide additional benefit in some. Both agents are considered to have modest central pain modulating properties. In severe cases, patients may require intravesical heparin, which involves squirting heparin into the bladder. The patient self-administers heparin mixed in water into the bladder. How heparin works to relieve symptoms is unknown. Interstitial cystitis frequently requires the use of combination therapy to improve functional outcome. Referral for psychological evaluation and appropriate intervention may be indicated. Psychological intervention should focus on helping the patient develop more effective coping strategies and pain management skills, such as relaxation and distraction techniques. Cognitive and behavioral therapies can be effective in reducing depressive symptoms and managing pain.

### Sickle Cell Disease

If there is one word to describe the life of patients with sickle cell disease, it is "painful." Sickle cell disease involves recurrent episodes of acute pain and pain associated with resulting tissue damage. One of every 375 African Americans has sickle cell anemia. This is an inherited blood disorder in which structurally abnormal hemoglobin is present and results in sickling (breakdown) of the red blood cells. This leads to problems in the vessels and tissues. The red cells change shape from round and smooth to spiked and rigid. They can no longer squeeze through narrow blood vessels, and they form plugs and disrupt circulation to tissues, which is the source of the pain. People with this disease used to die at a young age, but now with better treatments patients may live into their adult years.

Painful episodes are unpredictable, recurrent, and intense and frequently lead to emergency room visits and hospitalizations. As with many painful conditions, nonopiate analgesics and opiate analgesics form the foundation of pain management, since the intensity of pain tends to be severe in these patients. Other measures include rehydration, oxygen to preserve tissue health, and psychological support.

### Treatment

In a given year, about 60 percent of patients with sickle cell disease will experience an episode of severe pain. Hospital personnel do not always recognize sickle cell disease as a chronic disorder and may not be adequately educated about the disease and its associated problems. Patients may feel stereotyped as opiate dependent or drug seeking, and they may become distrustful and apprehensive of medical services. Hence, they may postpone treatment until a crisis has become severe. Addressing the pain with oral analgesic drugs that the patient may take at home can reduce length of hospital stay and number of admissions, as well as improving quality of life, incidentally cutting costs substantially. Prescribing oral analgesics appropriately may be a matter of educating health care providers as well as the patient and family. Early aggressive treatment of a crisis pain episode is necessary. One barrier in achieving early effective therapy may be the lack of social support networks and education, especially for indigent patients.

While narcotic pain medications are the mainstay, new therapies are available that reduce the frequency of painful crises. These include hydroxyurea, which is helpful in approximately one-third of the patient population. Magnesium and clotrimazole both help prevent dehydration, and nitric oxide may help damaged blood vessels. A specific problem called "priapism" is prolonged painful penile engorgement. Recently, an outpatient procedure done under local anesthetic has reportedly reversed this painful episode in several sickle cell patients. This procedure includes penile aspiration and epinephrine irrigation.

Patients with severe pain should be given pain medications at frequent, fixed intervals until the pain has diminished. Some patients can be given oral analgesic drugs such as Tylenol with codeine for mild to moderate pain. Nonsteroidal anti-inflammatory drugs can be used for bone pain. For chronic, severe pain, fentanyl patches (Duragesic) can be useful. Opiates such as meperidine (Demerol) are controversial in these patients in crisis. Demerol has a metabolite normeperidine, a brain irritant that is excreted through the kidneys. This compound may accumulate and cause serious side effects, including seizures.

Using placebo formulations to evaluate the severity of painful episodes is unethical and hinders the relationship between patient and health care provider. Conflicting perceptions between patients and staff about pain that is reported and analgesia that is required probably contribute most to poor pain management in sickle cell disease. Patients sometimes develop severe pain and other symptoms that require immediate medical attention. When seen in hospital emergency rooms, patients are often treated by physicians and nurses who may not know their case histories and who may assume, particularly if these medical personnel are unfamiliar with the treatment of sickle cell, that a patient is drug seeking. This can result in the undertreatment of serious pain. To prevent this problem, the patient or family should attempt to contact the treating physician. Additionally, a record of medications and pharmacies should be maintained and brought to the emergency room, along with containers of all prescription drugs. If there are frequent episodes requiring after-hours medical services because of acute pain episodes, the treating physician should be advised. Reevaluation of the patient's medication regimen may be needed and may indicate a need for additional opiate medications for breakthrough pain.

### Headaches

Headaches are one of the most common physical problems people experience. *Mal de tête*, the French term for headache, literally means pain in the head. Head pain can range from being mildly annoying to being severe and frequent in occurrence. Sleep can be disturbed, and daily activities can be difficult to perform. Headaches commonly have an origin in structures surrounding the brain, rather than coming from the brain itself. For example, the bones of the skull lack pain sensation, and the meninges, or lining tissues of the skull, are sensitive only in certain areas. The brain itself is very insensitive; on the other hand, the sinuses of the brain are very sensitive.

More than 45 million Americans experience some form of headache on a recurrent basis. Chronic headache sufferers spend $2.5 to $4 billion each year on treatments. Today, the causes of headaches are better understood, and there are many treatment options available to effectively control head pain in most patients.

While most headaches are not associated with a serious condition, in some cases head pain can be serious and require immediate medical attention. A physician should be consulted if the headache is accompanied by confusion, unconsciousness, or convulsions. Medical consultation should also be sought if an individual sustains a blow to the head or if head pain becomes persistent in an individual who was previously free of headaches. Other danger signals include pain in the eye or ear and headache accompanied by fever and nausea. The majority of headaches are a result of tension. These headaches are frequently described as feeling like the tightening of a band around the head, a sensation that is worse during times of increased stress or muscle tension. Cluster headaches are acute attacks of severe, one-sided head pain that last from a few minutes to a few hours. These attacks can occur daily for four to twelve weeks. One to three episodes can occur daily, even during sleep. Between attacks the patient is usually pain free. Cluster headaches are accompanied by other symptoms such as excess tearing or facial flushing, and are most common in men.

Migraines are also called vascular headaches, because they are associated with changes in the blood vessels of the brain. An estimated 23 million Americans suffer disabling migraines. These headaches may begin in childhood, but almost always develop before the age of thirty. Approximately 60 to 70 percent of migraine sufferers are female. Sixteen percent of these patients experience head pain severe enough to warrant medical attention. An estimated 150 million workdays are lost annually because of migraines, at an estimated cost of $6 to $17 billion.

Migraines are periodic unilateral headaches that may be classified into categories according to the history given by the patient. Common migraine (nonclassic) is a headache occurring without neurologic warning symptoms. This accounts for about 85 percent of all migraines. In classic migraine, distinctive neurologic signs occur in the few minutes preceding the onset of headache pain and are termed "aura." These signs are likely a result of changes in the circulation of the brain. Substance P may be one agent responsible for transmitting these changes and registering them as pain. Attacks may be triggered by any number of factors such as perfumes, alcohol, or cheddar cheese. The warning signs of an aura may include such symptoms as flashing lights, numbness in the arms, dizziness, nausea, or other neurological disturbances.

Since migraines occur more often in women than in men, hormones may play a role in triggering migraine attacks. Approximately 60 percent of women relate the onset of migraines to their menstrual cycle. Also, genetics may predispose individuals to this condition. Often there is a family history of migraines or headaches.

### Treatment

Treatment of headaches may take several different forms directed toward treating the acute event or preventing further episodes. Multiple medications are often tried, as well as behavioral modifications. The combination of stress management and tension reduction, with regular daily exercise and stretching, can be an effective method of prevention. Medical therapy begins with milder analgesics, while headache-specific medications are used in patients with more severe symptoms.

Treatment of tension headaches usually includes psychological interventions directed toward reducing stress. Physical therapy to decrease muscle tension may also be helpful. Cluster headaches are acute events and are best managed with specific therapy. Oxygen administered by mask in 100 percent concentration may break a cluster headache within minutes. Steroids are required by some, especially if oxygen is not a practical treatment. Lithium and several other medications are occasionally tried.

Migraine-specific medications fall into categories such as ergotamines and triptans. Ergotamines are used to treat severe, throbbing head pain that can occur in migraine and cluster headaches. However, they relieve only the throbbing pain and do not relieve other types of pain and symptoms. Additionally, rebound headaches may occur from the ergotamines if they are used for more than two days. Triptans are sometimes preferred because they relieve associated symptoms such as nausea and light sensitivity as well as the headache pain. They are also called "abortives," as they are taken to abort the headache symptoms. Four of these drugs that have received FDA approval are sumatriptan (Imitrex), zolmitriptan (Zomig), naratriptan (Amerge), and rizatriptan (Maxalt). Treatment is sometimes aimed at preventing recurrences of headaches or decreasing their frequency. Medications are usually titrated over one to three months until the frequency of the headaches decreases. The vascular or blood flow component is treated with blood pressure medications such as beta blockers or calcium channel blockers. The recent discovery of a mutation in a brain calcium-channel gene in families with hemiplegic migraines (symptoms of facial paralysis) and in families with episodic vertigo and ataxia suggests a possible mechanism for neurotologic symptoms (motion sickness, vertigo, noise sensitivity) in patients with more common varieties of migraine. A defective calcium channel, primarily expressed in the brain and inner ear, is thought to lead to reversible hair cell changes and auditory and vestibular symptoms.

Antiepileptic agents may also be useful in preventing some refractory migraines. Nonsteroidal anti-inflammatory drugs have been shown to be effective in some migraine patients. Tricyclic antidepressants are most useful in tension-type headaches, but may also be tried in refractory, difficult-to-control migraines. No one therapy works in all patients. Individual considerations are necessary, as there is a wide variability in effectiveness of treatments. Despite these limitations, most patients can be helped.

# 10. The Search for Cures

Hope, the patent medicine. . . .

—Wallace Rice

Although we have found no cure for chronic pain, we have come a long, long way. The observations made by Bonica and Livingston of pain in injured soldiers during World War II influenced their recognition of pain as a multifactorial phenomenon and motivated their establishment of the first interdisciplinary treatment centers. Melzack and Wall followed with the publication of the gate control theory of pain in 1965. These events have generated much research over the last two decades and have led to the application of a multimodality model in the assessment and treatment of chronic pain. With these achievements the importance of the biopsychosocial model of disease has been underscored in our search for a greater understanding of chronic pain mechanisms and factors that influence pain and suffering.

Psychosocial variables have a significant role in the pain experience, and there appears to be a neurological basis for observed psychological phenomena. The influence of a descending pathway in the modulation of pain perception is generally accepted. With the progress made, a shift has occurred in our thinking about chronic pain. Chronic pain is no longer just considered a symptom of disease or injury or necessarily psychogenic in origin but is recognized as a separate and distinct disease state worthy of scientific investigation and clinical treatment in its own right. We have

transcended many barriers, and through these efforts the
pain and suffering experienced by millions of individuals have
been legitimized
      As we have seen, pain is now accepted as the fifth vital
sign. This concept was created by the American Pain Society
in 1995 to increase awareness among health care professionals
that pain should be addressed and treated. Increased public
and professional education has brought the importance of
pain treatment to the forefront. In 1999 the Joint Commission
on Accreditation of Health care Organizations (JCAHO)
announced the development and approval of standards that
created new requirements for the assessment and management
of pain in accredited hospitals and other health care settings.
These standards are included in the 2000–2001 standards
manual. JCAHO clearly acknowledges that pain is a condition
coexisting with many other diseases and injuries and that it
requires specific attention and intervention. Currently, efforts
to influence public policy and legislation, increase public education, and generate increased funding for research are under
way in many states and on a federal level. Organizations such
as the American Pain Society, the International Association
for the Study of Pain, and patient advocacy groups strongly
support education, treatment, and research.
      Research is typically conducted through a series of clinical
trials. A clinical trial is a study designed to answer specific
questions about potential new therapies or new ways of using known treatments. Clinical trials are used to determine
whether new drugs or treatments are both safe and effective.
All clinical trials are based on a set of rules called a protocol.
A protocol describes what types of people may participate in
the trial; the schedule of tests, procedures, medications, and
dosages; and the length of the study. Clinical trials are conducted by government agencies, pharmaceutical companies,
health care institutions, organizations that develop medical
devices or equipment, and individual investigators hired by
such groups. Trials can take place in a variety of locations,

such as hospitals, universities, physician offices, or outpatient clinics.

Clinical trials on experimental drugs are usually conducted in four phases. Phase I clinical trials test a new drug or treatment in a small group of people for the first time to evaluate its safety, determine a safe dosage range, and identify side effects. The second phase involves a larger group of people, and phase III trials expand the testing to include even more. Phase III trials often involve thousands of people and can last for several years. These studies provide researchers with a thorough understanding of the drug's effectiveness, its benefits, and the range of possible side effects. Once phase III testing is successfully completed, the sponsor will request Federal Drug Administration (FDA) approval for marketing of the drug. In phase IV the long-term benefits of the drug are evaluated, and studies may be conducted comparing the cost-effectiveness of the drug to traditional treatments.

All studies have guidelines about who can participate. Guidelines are based on factors such as age, type of disease, medical history, and current medical condition. Interested persons can get information about clinical trials by contacting local medical centers, pharmaceutical companies, pain organizations, and the National Institutes of Health (NIH) and by using Web sites such as ClinicalTrials.gov (sponsored by NIH) or DrugStudyCentral.com. The NIH Web site provides information on clinical trials currently recruiting participants and tells you who to contact.

Currently, researchers are attempting to answer questions about the basic mechanisms of pain through investigation of pain receptors, ion channels, neuroplasticity, molecular genetics, neurotransmitters, and specific brain structures involved in pain processing. These efforts are leading to the development of new treatments and drug therapies and are helping us understand why certain interventions are effective in decreasing pain. We are also gaining insight into the individual variability of pain among patients and are looking toward developing specific treatments for specific pain disorders tailored for specific patient populations.

Positron emission tomography (PET) and magnetic resonance imaging (MRI) are being used to identify areas of the brain activated by pain. We know that pain is a unified experience with discriminative, affective-motivational, and cognitive components. Each of these factors is mediated through forebrain mechanisms acting at spinal, brainstem, and cerebral levels. Animal models and human imaging studies are helping increase our understanding of forebrain mechanisms of normal and pathological pain. The first success in capturing a still image of pain in the brain was reported in 1991 by Dr. Jeanne Talbot of the University of Montreal and Dr. Catherine Bushnell of McGill University. They used PET scanning to watch pain centers in the brain as messages were processed and transmitted by nerve cells at the site of injury. Four regions of the brain were identified as important in the sensing of pain: the primary and secondary somatosensory cortices, the anterior cingulate cortex, insular cortex, and regions of the frontal cortex. Further studies by Dr. Bushnell and colleagues found evidence strongly supporting a prominent role for the primary somatosensory cortex in the sensory aspects of pain, including localization and discrimination of pain intensity.

Another imaging study led by Dr. Kenneth Casey at the University of Michigan used an animal model to investigate areas of the brain activated by pain. Results showed a progressive and selective activation of somatosensory and limbic system structures in the brain and brainstem following injection of formalin (pain-producing substance) into a rat's paw. The National Institute of Dental and Craniofacial Research (NIDCR) is currently sponsoring somatosensory studies of pain and pain control measured with PET scanning and functional MRI in patients with neuropathic and chronic pain. Research in these areas may lead to the identification of new pain pathways, a greater understanding of pain processing in different chronic pain conditions, and more objective methods of measuring pain.

Neuroplasticity is the ability of neurons to alter their structure and function in response to internal and external stimuli. It is believed that physical and chemical neuroplastic changes occur with learning, memory, and chronic pain. Preliminary evidence suggests that if severe pain persists, neuroplastic changes related to the development of incurable chronic pain syndromes begin to take place. However, even after the onset of chronic pain conditions, cognitions and behaviors can be learned which may serve to restore more adaptive physiological, cognitive, and behavioral patterns. Currently, methods are available that allow scientists to study these changes and nervous system reorganization that occur during the processing of pain.

Neurotrophins, usually proteins, facilitate growth and repair of nerve cells and are thought to be involved in hyperalgesia. Certain receptors found on cells respond to trophic factors and interact with each other. Studies have shown that some trophic compounds can reverse changes in neurons after injury, possibly producing a decrease in pain sensation, while others serve to heighten pain sensitivity. The investigation of neurotrophins and how they interact could lead to new pain interventions. At times neurons in the pain pathway overreact to painful and sometimes nonpainful stimuli. The process, triggered by inflammation or tissue injury, is partly mediated by a neurotrophin, nerve growth factor (NGF), which causes pain-sensing neurons to react more readily to noxious stimuli.

Dr. Lorne Mendell of the State University of New York at Stony Brook found evidence that NGF may enhance the response of sensory neurons by increasing the activity of the capsaicin receptors. Another trophic factor was recently identified by a group of researchers in London. Brain-derived neurotrophin factor (BDNF) released from nociceptive terminals may contribute to sensory abnormalities associated with some pathophysiological states, such as inflammatory conditions. Preliminary data suggests that blocking BDNF at least partially prevents some aspects of pain development (central sensitization).

Recently, many advances in molecular genetics have been made. Certain genetic mutations are believed to change pain sensitivity and behavioral responses to pain. Disruptions or changes are caused in the processing of pain information as it leaves the spinal cord and travels to the brain. Additionally, researchers are beginning to understand why individuals experience pain differently. Although the relative importance of genetic influences versus experience in human pain perception is unclear, animal research is demonstrating possible genetic differences in both nociceptive and analgesic sensitivity. Scientists are predicting that within the next ten years it will be possible to collect DNA and analyze it for common genetic variations associated with various diseases. This may lead to the early identification, prevention, and treatment of potential chronic disease states, thus preventing the development of chronic pain that is secondary to specific disease and uncovering the basis of genetic influences on pain perception.

Dr. Jeffrey Mogil, assistant professor of psychology at the University of Illinois, is conducting studies to identify specific genes responsible for response to pain. Mogil found that certain strains of mice are more sensitive to pain, and these strains are less responsive to analgesics such as morphine. Also, involved genes are different in males and females, resulting in neurochemical differences. The National Institute of Dental and Craniofacial Research is currently sponsoring a phase II study concerned with the role of genetics in pain sensitivity. The study will investigate genetic contributions to acute experimental pain and clinical postoperative pain. In the future, research may allow health care practitioners to assess and treat pain on an individual basis. It may also help us understand why some people are more sensitive to pain than others, and eliminate the stigma attached to those individuals.

A recent study conducted by Dr. George Uhl and colleagues at Johns Hopkins University demonstrated that differences in pain perception are also due to a variation on the surface of nerve cells of a molecule called the mu opiate receptor. Studies of humans and mice show that the number of these receptors directly affects the sensitivity to pain, and that the receptors, in turn, are linked to a single gene called the mu opiate receptor gene. The mu receptor works by bonding with natural chemicals called peptides that help diminish the sensation of pain. When lots of receptors are present, the perception of pain is diminished. However, when there are fewer receptors or none at all, the nerve cell takes up fewer peptides, and even a small stimulus is perceived as painful. The mu receptor is the primary target of some opiate drugs that help control severe pain. Researchers may discover how to identify genetically the level of opiates each patient will need to control pain.

In studies of neurotransmitters and pain receptors, evidence is suggesting distinct neurochemistries for acute and chronic pain. This points to the likelihood that chronic pain is a disease state of the nervous system and not merely a prolonged acute pain symptom of other disease conditions. Receptors have been identified which may play a role in specific types of chronic pain disorders. For example, capsaicin, which is derived from chili peppers and is used to study pain physiology, causes a sensation of burning pain by selectively activating sensory neurons that send messages about noxious stimuli to the central nervous system. Dr. David Julius and Dr. John Levine of the University of California, San Francisco (UCSF) cloned the capsaicin receptor that is found exclusively in pain-processing neurons. They found that when capsaicin binds to its receptor, it opens a channel and excites the neuron, which then transmits its pain signal. The same receptors are also on neurons activated by heat. Levine and colleagues found that overstimulating the receptor can reduce clinical pain. Decreasing certain pain sensations may be possible by inactivating or altering this process. The capsaicin receptor is among the first molecular markers for delineating nociceptors. His group named the receptor VRI, after an essential chemical component of capsaicin. Researchers at SmithKline Beecham are now screening compounds for their effects on VRI.

Investigators are also exploring the role of ion channels in pain processing. Sodium channels, in general, control the excitability of neurons all over the body. However, pain-sensing neurons have been found to have a unique type of sodium channel. Dr. John Wood's research at the University College in London and Dr. John Hunter and colleagues at Roche Bioscience in Palo Alto identified a sodium channel found almost exclusively in small diameter pain-sensing neurons. This channel, named PN3, is unusual in that it is resistant to tetrodotoxin (TTX), a neurotoxin from puffer fish that disables many other sodium channels.

Roche researchers examined the distribution of PN3 in neurons following nerve injury in rats, which is a model for human neuropathic pain. They found that PN3 accumulates at the site of injury. Regarding exaggerated sensitivity (sensitization), they hypothesized that perhaps the redistribution changes the sensitivity of the neuron, causing it to respond inappropriately to stimuli that would normally not be considered painful. Roche and other pharmaceutical companies are involved in research to find inhibitors that will selectively block the activation of this TTX-resistant sodium channel, leaving other TTX-sensitive channels functioning normally.

Another TTX-resistant sodium channel, SNS2, was identified by Dr. Clifford Woolf and his colleagues at the Massachusetts General Hospital in collaboration with Glaxo Wellcome in England. The sodium channel is found exclusively in pain neurons. They are working toward understanding whether it has a specific role in pain transmission. Additionally, Dr. Woolf and researchers at other facilities are attempting to develop a mouse strain lacking one or both genes, to determine which, if either, sodium channel might be central to pain transmission.

Dr. Allan Basbaum of UCSF and Dr. Susumu Tonegawa at the Massachusetts Institute of Technology genetically engineered a mouse that lacks a particular form of a signaling molecule called protein kinase-C (PKC). When neurons carrying pain messages are excited, their channels open and calcium floods into the cells. Calcium influx activates molecules, including PKC, that transmit pain signals. The researchers hypothesized that by eliminating or blocking PKC pain might be reduced. Results of preliminary studies show that mice without PKC respond normally to acute pain, but the mice fail to develop the neuropathic pain syndrome seen in normal mice when their sciatic nerves are injured.

As we gain a greater understanding of the basic physiology and the mechanisms involved in chronic pain, pain-relieving drugs can be developed that target specific sites. Recent results from studies led by Dr. Richard Pellegrino from Central Arkansas Research, Inc., appear promising regarding a new drug for the treatment of nighttime pain associated with diabetic peripheral neuropathy. Memantine targets the N-methyl-D-aspartate (NMDA) receptor implicated in the development of secondary hyperalgesia involved with somatic, neural, and visceral structures. By blocking this receptor, decreases in neuropathic pain have been shown in some patients. A phase III trial is under way.

Other current studies include a phase II trial that will investigate the effectiveness of a new drug, flecainide, in treating patients with chronic neuropathic pain from cancer or AIDS. Sponsored by the National Cancer Institute (NCI), clinical trials will be conducted in several locations that include the Veterans Affairs Medical Center in Madison, Wisconsin, and the Riverview Medical Center in Red Bank, New Jersey.

The National Institute of Dental and Craniofacial Research will sponsor a study to evaluate the effects of the drug

LY293558 on pain perception in patients with neuropathic pain. During the last several years, there has been increasing evidence suggesting that chronic pain due to nerve or soft tissue injury may result in sensitization of the central nervous system, and is modulated by the excitatory amino acids, glutamate, and aspartate. The development of compounds which both excite and block the three classes of receptors to which excitatory amino acids bind has led to data which suggest that a new therapeutic approach is to directly block excitation. LY293558 is considered a receptor blocker and may be effective in altering pain perception.

Researchers funded by the National Institute of Neurological Disorders and Stroke (NINDS) are working toward reducing sensitivity to stimuli associated with chronic neuropathic and inflammatory pain by disabling certain nerve cells that send pain signals to the brain. At the University of Minnesota investigators found that by injecting a combination of substance P (a neurotransmitter known to stimulate pain receptors) and SAP (the ribosome-inactivating protein saporin) into the dorsal horn of the spinal cord in rats, there is a lessened pain response to thermal and mechanically induced pain following nerve injury, inflammation, and the long-term effects of pain produced by capsaicin injection. Additionally, it was shown that substance P-SAP treatment reduced the number of spinal cord neurons that express substance P receptor. Researchers are now looking toward performing toxicology studies in large animals to demonstrate the safety and efficacy of this treatment in another species. If these studies are successful, approval will be sought to treat terminally ill cancer patients who have severe chronic pain to determine the extent of the relief of chronic pain in humans.

Neurotropin, a nonprotein extract of cutaneous tissue from rabbits inoculated with vaccinia virus, has been used extensively in Japan to treat reflex sympathetic dystrophy and other painful conditions. However, the drug has not undergone clinical testing in the United States. The National

Institute of Dental and Craniofacial Research will sponsor a phase II trial to determine the clinical efficacy of Neurotropin for treatment of acute pain in dental outpatients and for chronic pain in outpatients with reflex sympathetic dystrophy.

Abbott Pharmaceuticals is sponsoring research on nicotine-based drugs. Nicotine or nicotine agonists may serve as nonopioid drugs to treat chronic pain. Research at Virginia Commonwealth University demonstrated that in animals nicotine is active in chronic pain, inflammation, and neuropathic pain. The data suggests that some nicotine receptors are involved in serotonin pathways, the brain stem, the thalamus, the cortex, and the spinal cord. One drug, ABT-594, is in phase II clinical trials. ABT-594, developed from the toxin of South American tree frogs, is the first drug of its kind and is reported to have many times the strength of morphine without the side effects associated with morphine. Researchers at the University of California, San Francisco, are currently investigating whether the drug is safe and effective in controlling pain associated with diabetic neuropathy.

Many other drug studies are being conducted and are in various phases of clinical trials. Dr. Jack Rosenberg and colleagues at the University of Michigan Pain Clinic are currently studying the effects and efficacy of chronic narcotic treatment for nonmalignant pain. In another study funded by the National Cancer Institute researchers are evaluating the efficacy of two formulations of morphine in patients requiring morphine for the treatment of chronic cancer pain. Different drug formulations and combinations of drugs may help patients with chronic pain live more comfortably. However, it is not yet known which regimen is most effective for chronic pain.

Pharmacia, Inc., is sponsoring research on Parecoxib, the first investigational injectable COX-2 specific inhibitor. A recent study found that this drug was more effective for postsurgical pain than injectable morphine and a different NSAID. Further studies are investigating the potential use of Parecoxib for other pain conditions. Another pharmaceutical company, AstraZeneca, is in phase II trials of LEF, a peripherally acting opiate, for relief of acute and chronic pain. The company is also conducting a phase II trial to assess the efficacy of LTA, a sodium channel blocker, for analgesia.

For many years, researchers have worked toward identifying psychological, behavioral, and environmental factors involved in the pain experience. Through this research, we now know that many nonintrusive interventions, such as relaxation, may alter neurochemical and neurophysiological processes and serve to mediate pain. Many cognitive and behavioral therapies target misperceptions about pain and assist patients in reconceptualizing their condition and the impact it has on their lives. Additionally, these therapies may affect treatment outcome associated with other therapeutic interventions. For example, patient expectations and pain perceptions can play an important role in determining the effectiveness of many interventions. Part of the effectiveness or failure of drug therapies and other treatments can be attributed to patient expectations or a placebo response.

Furthermore, studies are aimed at delineating other factors that affect treatment outcome. Environmental factors, such as the responses and attitudes of family members, employers, and health care providers, can affect patients' reactions to their pain. Job satisfaction and patients' perceptions of their condition (e.g., disabling vs. impairing, self-management of pain versus no pain control) are often predictors of a return to work for patients who have a low back pain disorder. A recent study at Ohio State University supported previous findings that psychological stress is linked to back pain and may increase the risk of work-related back injury. Research suggests that relaxation training, cognitive therapies, and biofeedback may be effective substitutes or adjuncts to medical treatments for chronic headache and low back pain.

Current cognitive-behavioral research includes projects sponsored by the National Cancer Institute (NCI) that will evaluate whether an outpatient educational and behavioral skills training program will improve pain control in patients with metastatic or recurrent breast or prostate cancer. It is hypothesized that cognitive-behavioral intervention may help patients live longer and improve the quality of their lives. In a study sponsored by the National Institute of Arthritis and Musculoskeletal and Skin Diseases (NIAMS), Dr. Dennis Turk at the University of Washington, Department of Anesthesiology, is the principal investigator evaluating the benefit of matching treatments to subject characteristics in patients with fibromyalgia. Treatment protocols will include a standardized physical therapy program and either cognitive-behavioral pain management therapy, interpersonal skill training, or supportive counseling. Dr. Jack Edinger and colleagues at the Veterans Administration Medical Center-Brooklyn in Durham, North Carolina, will test the effectiveness of a nondrug treatment for insomnia that often accompanies fibromyalgia. Specifically, a cognitive-behavioral therapy previously shown to be effective in treating sleep disturbance will be evaluated.

In our efforts toward developing better treatments and ultimately a cure for chronic pain, we must carry out a multilevel strategy. That is, we must continue to improve assessment and treatment regimens and incorporate education for family members, social support systems, and employers. Secondly, greater emphasis should be placed on pain education in health care training program curriculums and continuing education requirements. Policy makers should be informed about chronic pain and the importance of funding for treatment and research. Insurance companies and other third-party reimbursement entities should be educated about the efficacy of pain treatment and the cost-effectiveness of providing appropriate prevention and early intervention. Last, and most important, communication and cooperation among the many disciplines involved in research and treatment efforts are vital if these challenges are to be successfully met.

We now have a common philosophy and common language stretching across disciplines and allowing us to address the multifactorial nature of chronic pain. Currently, one of the most effective treatment models is an interdisciplinary team approach that recognizes the important role patients have in their treatment process and emphasizes the use of multiple interventions in combating the problem of pain. As we continue to gain insights, our treatments will become more effective, and we will be able to more clearly delineate specific treatment regimens for specific chronic pain conditions. We will also be able to define what works best for what patients. It is to those who truly believe that chronic pain is "real" that we extend our thanks and gratitude for their continued efforts toward alleviating the devastating consequences and suffering experienced by affected individuals.

For the millions who suffer from chronic pain, hope lies in the acknowledgment that chronic pain is "real." We have opened the door to a better understanding of the underlying mechanisms of chronic pain. This knowledge will lead us to formulate new questions and travel down new paths of discovery. Technological advances have enabled researchers to view the nervous system in greater detail and with more sophistication. One day, cures for chronic pain will be found. Meanwhile, treatment models and therapies are available that can be effective in managing chronic pain and can serve to help patients improve the quality of their lives.

# Appendix

The following organizations provide information and education about the management of chronic pain. The Web sites given are themselves informative and often are links to other pain education sites. Most of the Web sites listed under "Pain" offer information on many different chronic pain conditions.

## AIDS

CDC Division of HIV/AIDS Prevention
1600 Clifton Road, NE, M/S E-49
Atlanta, GA 30333
800/343-2437
Information: www.cdc.gov/hiv
Clinical trials: www.actis.org

## Back Pain

National Institute of Arthritis and Musculoskeletal and Skin
   Diseases (NIAMS)
Bethesda, MD 20892-2350
www.nih.gov

Spondylitis Association of America
14827 Ventura Blvd. #222
Sherman Oaks, CA 91403
800/777-8189
www.spondylitis.org

## Cancer

American Alliance of Cancer Pain Initiatives
1300 University Avenue
Madison, WI 53706
608/265-4013
www.aacpi.org

American Cancer Society
National Office
1599 Clifton Road, NE
Atlanta, GA 30329
800/ACS-2345
www.cancer.org

Cancer Care
275 7th Avenue
New York, NY 10001
800/813-4673
www.cancercare.org

National Cancer Institute
800/4-CANCER
www.nci.nih.gov

OncoLink
www.oncolink.com

Oncology Nursing Society
501 Holiday Drive
Pittsburgh, PA 15220-2749
412/921-7373
www.ons.org

Pegasus Education Technologies, Ltd.
936 Peace Portal Drive
Blaine, WA 98230
Distributes *The Living with Cancer Video Series Program for Indigent Patients on PO MS*
Contact: Roxane Laboratories, 800/848-0120
Purdue Frederick Co., 800/877-0123
Janssen (Duragesic), 800/544-2987

Purdue Frederick Co.
100 Connecticut Avenue
Norwalk, CT 06850-3590
800/877-0123
Distributes *My Word Against Theirs* (cancer pain videotapes) and *Home Care of the Hospice Patient* (patient/family education)

Resource Center for State Cancer Pain Initiatives
University of Wisconsin-Madison, Medical Sciences Center
1300 University Avenue
Madison, WI 53706
608/265-4013
www.wisc.edu/molpharm/wcpi

### Fibromyalgia

American Fibromyalgia Syndrome Association, Inc.
6380 E. Tanque Verde, Suite D
Tucson, AZ 85715
520/733-1570
www.afsafund.org

## Head Pain

American Council for Headache Education (ACHE)
19 Mantua Road
Mount Royal, NJ 08061
856/423-0258
www.achenet.org

Migraine Information Center
JAMA Migraine Information Center
www.ama-assn.org/special/migraine/support/support.htm

National Headache Foundation
428 W. St. James Place, 2nd Fl.
Chicago, IL 60614-2750
888/NHF-5552
www.headaches.org

## Interstitial Cystitis

Interstitial Cystitis Association
51 Monroe Street, Suite 1402
Rockville, MD 20850
301/610-5300
www.ichelp.com

## Nerve Pain

American Diabetes Association
1701 North Beauregard St.
Alexandria, VA 22311
800/342-2383
www.diabetes.org

National Institute of Dental and Craniofacial Research
  (NIDCR)
www.nidr.nih.gov

National Institute of Neurological Disorders and Stroke
  (NINDS)
P.O. Box 5801
Bethesda, MD 20824
www.ninds.nih.gov

The Neuropathy Association
60 E. 42nd Street, Suite 942
New York, NY 10165-5714
212/692-0662
www.neuropathy.org

Reflex Sympathetic Dystrophy Syndrome Association of
  America
P.O. Box 502
Milford, CT 06460
203/877-3790
www.rsds.org

Trigeminal Neuralgia Association
P.O. Box 340
Barnegat Light, NJ 08006
609/361-1014
www.tna-support.org

**Pain**

American Academy of Pain Management
13947 Monoway #A
Sonora, CA 95370
209/533-9744
www.aapainmanage.org

American Academy of Pain Medicine
4700 W. Lake Avenue
Glenview, IL 60025
847/375-4731
www.painmed.org

American Chronic Pain Association
P.O. Box 850
Rocklin, CA 95677
916/632-0922
www.theacpa.org

American Pain Foundation
III S. Calvert Street, Suite 2700
Baltimore, MD 21202
www.painfoundation.org

American Pain Society
4500 West Lake Avenue
Glenview, IL 60025-1485
847/375-4715
www.ampainsoc.org

International Association for the Study of Pain
909 NE 43rd Street, Suite 306
Seattle, WA 98105-6020
206/547-6409
www.halcyon.com/iasp

Medtronic
www.medtronic.com

National Chronic Pain Outreach Association
7979 Old Georgetown Road, Suite 100
Bethesda, MD 20814-2429
301/652-4948

The National Foundation for the Treatment of Pain
1330 Skyline Drive, #21
Monterey, CA 93940
831/655-8812
www.paincare.org

Pain.com
www.pain.com

Partners Against Pain
www.partnersagainstpain.com

Roxane Pain Institute
P.O. Box 16532
Columbus, OH 43216-6532
800/335-9100
www.roxane.com

### Rheumatic Pain

Arthritis Foundation
P.O. Box 7669
Atlanta, GA 30357-0669
404/872-7100
www.arthritis.org

National Institute of Arthritis and Musculoskeletal and Skin
    Diseases (NIAMS)
301/496-8190
www.nih.gov

National Osteoporosis Foundation
1232 22nd Street, NW
Washington, DC 20037-1292
202/223-2226
www.nof.org

**Sickle Cell Pain**

Sickle Cell Disease Association of America, Inc.
200 Corporate Pointe, Suite 495
Culver City, CA 90230-8727
800/421-8453
www.sicklecelldisease.org

Sickle Cell Information Center
P.O. Box 109
Grady Memorial Hospital
80 Butler Street SE
Atlanta, GA 30303
404/616-3572
www.emory.edu/PEDS/SICKLE/

# Glossary

**Action potential** An impulse that travels down an axon when sodium rushes into the cell and the neuron becomes depolarized. This kind of nerve communication is "all or none": the cell either fires at full strength or does not fire at all.

**Allodynia** Pain that results from a noninjurious stimulus to the skin.

**Analgesia** Absence of pain in response to stimulation that would normally be painful.

**Anesthesia** Total or partial loss of sensation, especially tactile sensibility, induced by disease, injury, acupuncture, or an anesthetic.

**Anesthetic** An agent that produces regional anesthesia (in one part of the body) or general anesthesia (loss of consciousness).

**Axon** The usually long process of a nerve fiber that generally conducts impulses away from the body of the nerve cell.

**Biofeedback** A training technique that enables a person to gain some voluntary control over autonomic body functions. It is based on the principle that a desired response is learned when received information indicates that a specific thought or action has produced such a response.

**Breakthrough pain** Intermittent exacerbations of pain that can occur spontaneously or in relation to specific activity.

**Bursa** A sac of fluid near the joint that lubricates the movement of muscles.

**Cartilage** The tough material that cushions and protects the ends of the bones and is also found in other parts of the body, such as the outer ear, larynx, and nose.

**Central pain** Pain associated with a lesion of the central nervous system.

**Cerebral cortex** The extensive outer layer of gray matter of the cerebral hemispheres, largely responsible for higher brain functions, including sensation, voluntary muscle movement, thought, reasoning, and memory.

**Chemotherapy** The treatment of disease with chemical agents or drugs that are selectively toxic to the causative agent or diseased tissue (cancer cells).

**Cognitive reappraisal** A coping strategy in which patients are taught to monitor and evaluate negative thoughts and replace them with more positive thoughts and images.

**Cordotomy** Surgery to cut some of the fibers of the spinal cord; used to relieve severe pain.

**Dendrite** In a neuron, the fiber that receives signals from the axons of other neurons and carries that signal to the cell body. A neuron can have up to several thousand dendrites.

**Deoxyribonucleic acid (DNA)** The chemical inside the nucleus of a cell that carries the genetic instructions for making living organisms. Each DNA molecule consists of two strands of sugar, phosphate, and nitrogen-containing molecules twisted around each other in a double spiral.

**Dermatome** An area of skin innervated by sensory fibers from a single spinal nerve.

**Distraction** The cognitive strategy of focusing attention on stimuli other than pain or negative emotions that accompany pain.

**Drug addiction** Pattern of compulsive drug use characterized by a continued craving for an opioid and the need to use the opioid for effects other than pain relief; psychological or emotional dependence on the effects of a drug.

**Drug tolerance** The decreasing effect of a drug with the same dose or the need to increase the dose to maintain the same effect.

**Dysesthesia** Impairment of sensation, especially that of touch, or a condition in which unpleasant sensation is produced by ordinary stimuli.

**Endorphin** One of a class of neurotransmitters that can bind to the same receptors that opiates such as morphine and heroin bind to and that produces the same behavioral effects of pain relief, euphoria, and, in high doses, sleep. Endorphins reduce the sensation of pain and affect emotions.

**Epidural** Situated within the spinal canal, on or outside the dura mater (tough membrane surrounding the spinal cord).

**Forebrain** The most highly developed part of the brain, responsible for the most complex aspects of behavior and mental life.

**Gate theory** An explanation of how the nervous system controls the amount of pain that reaches the brain. It holds that there is a functional "gate" in the spinal cord that either lets pain impulses travel to the brain or blocks their progress. Blocking occurs either when other sensations are let through instead of the pain impulses or when signals are sent down the spinal cord to close the gate.

**Hyperalgesia** Extreme sensitivity to pain.

**Hypnosis** A state of heightened awareness and focused concentration that can be used to manipulate the perception of pain.

**Imagery** A cognitive-behavioral strategy that uses mental images as an aid to relaxation and pain relief.

**Joint capsule** The sac that surrounds the cartilage.

**Lancinating** Characterized by piercing or stabbing sensations.

**Ligament** A band or sheet of tough fibrous tissue connecting two or more bones, cartilages, or other structures, or serving as support for muscles.

**Metastasis** The spread of cancer from one part of the body to another.

**Myelin** A fatty substance that wraps around some axons and increases the speed of action potentials.

**Myofascial pain** A large group of muscle disorders characterized by the presence of hypersensitive points, called trigger points, within one or more muscles and/or the investing connective tissue together with a syndrome of pain, muscle spasm, tenderness, stiffness, limitation of motion, weakness, and occasionally autonomic dysfunction.

**Nerve block** Pain relief method in which an anesthetic is injected into a nerve.

**Neuralgia** Pain in distribution of nerve or nerves.

**Neuron** The fundamental unit of the nervous system; a nerve cell, which has the ability to communicate with other nerve cells.

**Neuropathic pain/neuropathy** Pain that results from a disturbance of function or pathologic change in a nerve—in one nerve, mononeuropathy; in several nerves, mononeuropathy multiplex; if diffuse and bilateral, polyneuropathy.

**Neurotransmitter** Any of various chemical substances that transmit nerve impulses across a synapse.

**Nociceptor** A sensory receptor that responds to pain.

**Nonsteroidal anti-inflammatory drug (NSAID)** Aspirin-like drug that reduces inflammation (and hence pain) arising from injured tissue.

**Noxious** Damaging to the tissues.

**Nucleus** The part of a neuron which carries the genetic information that determines what kind of cell it will be and then acts to direct that cell's functioning.

**Opiate** Pain-killing drug chemically related to opium; also called a narcotic.

**Opiate receptor** Any of various cell membrane receptors that can bind with morphine and other opiates; concentrations of such receptors are especially high in regions of the brain having pain-related functions.

**Pain** An unpleasant sensory and emotional experience associated with actual or potential tissue damage or described in terms of such damage (International Association for the Study of Pain).

**Pain tolerance level** The greatest intensity of a pain-causing stimulus that a subject is prepared to tolerate.

**Paresthesia** A sensation on the skin, such as burning, prickling, itching, or tingling, with no apparent physical cause.

**Perception** The process through which people take raw sensations from the environment and interpret them, using knowledge, experience, and understanding of the world, so that the sensations become meaningful experiences.

**Placebo** A physical or psychological treatment that contains no active ingredient but produces an effect because the person receiving it believes it will. Part of the effectiveness of drugs is attributed to placebo.

**Progressive muscle relaxation** A cognitive-behavioral strategy in which muscles are alternately tensed and then relaxed in a systematic fashion.

**Radiation therapy** Treatment of disease with radiation, especially by selective irradiation with x-rays or other ionizing radiation. Radiation therapy is used to kill cancer cells.

**Receptor** A molecular structure or site on the surface or interior of a cell that binds with substances such as hormones, drugs, or neurotransmitters.

**Relaxation** A state of relative freedom from both anxiety and skeletal muscle tension. Relaxation techniques are used to lessen tension, reduce anxiety, and manage pain.

**Reticular formation** A network of nuclei and fibers threaded throughout the hindbrain and the midbrain that is composed of cells not arranged in a well-defined form. This network is very important in altering the activity of the rest of the brain. It is thought to play a role in attention and sleep.

**Self-statement** Part of a method that involves instructing patients to substitute positive thoughts for such negative ones as "I can't stand this" or "How much longer will this go on?"

**Sensory cortex** The part of the cerebral cortex located in the parietal, occipital, and temporal lobes which receives stimulus information from the skin, eyes, and ears, respectively.

**Serotonin** A neurotransmitter used by serotonergic neurons, which are located in the hindbrain and forebrain, to regulate sleep, mood, and pain sensation.

**Somatosensory** Of or relating to the perception of sensory stimuli from the skin and internal organs; derived from the Greek word for "body."

**Subcutaneous** Located, found, or placed just beneath the skin; hypodermic.

**Suffering** A state of severe distress associated with events that threaten the biological and/or psychological integrity of the individual. Suffering often accompanies severe pain but can occur in its absence.

**Synovial membrane** The connective-tissue membrane that lines the cavity of a synovial joint and produces the synovial fluid.

**Tendon** A band of tough, inelastic fibrous tissue that connects a muscle with its bony attachment.

**Thalamus** A brain structure in the forebrain that functions in the relay of sensory impulses to the cerebral cortex.

**Theory** An integrated set of principles that can be used to explain, predict, and control certain phenomena.

**Transcutaneous electrical nerve stimulation (TENS)** A method of producing electroanalgesia through electrodes applied to the skin.

**Trigger point** A specific point on the body at which touch or pressure will elicit pain.

# Index

Joint replacement, 33, 104, 106, 110.
 *See also* Arthroplasty

Kubler-Ross, Elisabeth, 61

Livingston, William K., 7, 128

Magnetic resonance imaging
 (MRI), 38, 79, 89, 131
Malingering, 80, 84
Manipulation, 50
Medications, 53–57
Melzack, Ronald, 7, 24, 26, 128
Migraine headaches, 33, 56, 125–27,
 146
Molecular genetics, 130, 133
Motor nerves, 89
Mu receptor, 134
Muscle relaxation, 47, 48
Myelin, 16, 88, 89
Myelograms, 38
Myofascial pain, 98–100
Myofascial release, 100

Narcotics, 5, 50, 121, 123, 138. *See
 also* Opiate Analgesics
National Cancer Institute (NCI),
 136, 138, 139, 144
National Institute of Arthritis
 and Musculoskeletal and Skin
 Diseases (NIAMS), 140, 143, 149
National Institute of Dental and
 Craniofacial Research (NIDCR),
 147
National Institute of Neurological
 Disorders and Stroke (NINDS),
 137, 147
Nerve conduction studies, 38, 89
Nerve entrapment, 90
Nerve growth factor (NGF), 132
Nerve pathways, 6, 13, 21
Neuralgia, 3

Neurons, 14–16
Neuropathic pain (nerve pain), 58,
 86, 88–97, 115, 135–38, 146–47
Neuroplasticity, 130, 132
Neurotoxin, 135
Neurotransmitters, 13, 16–18, 50, 130
Neurotrophins, 132
Nicotine, 138
N-methyl-D-aspartate (NMDA),
 136
Nociceptors, 22, 71, 116, 135
Nonopiate analgesics, 53–54, 122
Nonsteroidal Anti-inflammatory
 drugs (NSAIDs), 55–56
 degenerative disk, 73
 fibromyalgia, 102
 interstitial cystitis, 120
 migraine patients, 127
 osteoarthritis, 105
 postherpetic neuralgia, 93
 rheumatoid arthritis, 109
 sickle cell disease, 123
 spondyloarthropathies, 79
Norepinephrine, 56. *See also*
 Neurotransmitters

Opiate analgesics, 53, 54–55, 122,
 133
 fentanyl, 57, 86, 117, 123
 morphine, 6, 57, 113, 138
 morphine sulfate, 117
 oxycodone, 86, 117
Opium, 5, 6, 54
Osteoarthritis (OA), 35, 38, 99,
 103–06
Osteoporosis, 32, 37, 84
Osteotomy, 106

Pain
 behaviors, 84, 115
 cycle, 43, 49, 61, 63, 100
 definition of, 8–10

Understanding Health and Sickness Series
Miriam Bloom, Ph.D., General Editor

**Also in this series**

Addiction • Alzheimer's Disease • Anemia • Asthma • Childhood Obesity • Colon Cancer • Crohn Disease and Ulcerative
Colitis • Cystic Fibrosis • Dental Health • Depression • Hep-
atitis • Herpes • Panic and Other Anxiety Disorders • Sickle
Cell Disease

RB 127 .K645 2002

Koestler, Angela J.

Understanding chronic pain

DISCARDED BY

MACPHÁIDÍN LIBRARY

MACPHÁIDÍN LIBRARY
STONEHILL COLLEGE
EASTON, MASSACHUSETTS 02357